UNDERSTANDING LUPUS - NAVIGATING THE COMPLEXITIES OF AN AUTOIMMUNE JOURNEY

Dr. Bhratri Bhushan,
MD, DM

CONTENTS

PREFACE

Lupus is a word that comes with weight. For many, it arrives unexpectedly — sometimes after months or even years of mysterious symptoms, other times after a whirlwind of tests and doctor visits. No matter how it first enters your life, it rarely comes alone. It brings with it questions, fears, confusion, and uncertainty. It brings an endless search for answers in a world where even the experts don't always have them. And it brings the realization that life, as you once knew it, has changed.

This book was born out of the need to bridge the gap between medical knowledge and everyday life — between what doctors explain in hurried office visits and what patients actually need to understand to live well with lupus. Medical literature is full of facts about lupus, but for the person living with it day to day, facts are not enough. What's needed is guidance that makes sense in the context of real life — where symptoms fluctuate unpredictably, where medications come with side effects, where work, family, and personal dreams don't disappear just because a diagnosis has been made.

Lupus is often called the disease with a thousand faces, because it looks so different in each person it touches. Some live with mostly mild symptoms — joint pain, fatigue, skin rashes — while others face serious organ involvement requiring aggressive treatment. Some people have long stretches of remission, while others live in a constant push-pull between flares and recovery. There is no single roadmap that fits every person with lupus — but there is a way to build your own. This book is not about generic advice. It's about helping you understand your unique version of lupus, giving you the tools to track your patterns, understand your triggers, and develop your own personalized approach to care.

This book also recognizes something that's too often overlooked in medical conversations — lupus affects every part of you, not just your body. It affects your mental health, your relationships, your career, your sense of self. It asks you to redefine what strength means, not as pushing through pain, but as listening to your body and honoring its limits. It asks you to become an advocate for yourself in a healthcare system that doesn't always see invisible illnesses. It asks you to grieve what's been lost, while still building a meaningful and fulfilling life in the present.

Most of all, this book was written to remind you that you are not alone. Whether you were diagnosed yesterday or decades ago, whether your lupus is mild or severe, whether you've found a good rhythm or are still searching for answers — you are part of a community of warriors, each writing their own story, each facing the same frustrations, fears, and hopes.

Lupus may be unpredictable, but your approach to it doesn't have to be. With knowledge, compassion for yourself, and the right tools, you can become the expert on your own body, your own symptoms, and your own needs. This book is here to help you do that — to give you not just information, but understanding, strategies, and confidence.

This is not a book about how to fight lupus. It's a book about how to live with it — fully, bravely, and on your own terms. Welcome to your journey. Let's walk it together.

CHAPTER 1: UNDERSTANDING LUPUS: WHAT IS IT REALLY?

Lupus is a word many people have heard, but very few truly understand what it means, especially when they first encounter it. It often arrives with confusion, fear, and a long list of questions. What exactly is it? Is it contagious? Is it like cancer? Is it curable? There's a lot of misinformation out there, and the goal here is to take a step back and offer a clear, honest, and compassionate explanation of what lupus really is — without the intimidating medical language or unnecessary complexity. At its core, lupus is what doctors call an autoimmune disease. That simply means your immune system, which is supposed to protect you from infections and harmful invaders, gets confused and starts attacking your own healthy tissues instead. It's like a security system that can't tell the difference between a burglar and a family member. This mix-up causes inflammation, which is the body's way of reacting to injury or infection. In lupus, that inflammation can show up just about anywhere — skin, joints, kidneys, heart, lungs, brain, and even blood cells. This is why lupus is known as a systemic disease, meaning it can affect multiple organs and systems all at once or at different times.

Lupus is not a single disease with one clear shape.

It actually comes in several forms, and knowing the difference can help make sense of what you or your loved one is experiencing. The most common type, and the one people usually mean when they say "lupus," is systemic lupus erythematosus, often shortened to SLE. This is the form that can affect not just the skin and joints, but also internal organs like the kidneys, heart, and lungs. It's unpredictable, with symptoms that can flare up suddenly and then quiet down for a while, which is why it can feel so hard to get a handle on it. Then there's cutaneous lupus, which primarily affects the skin. Some people with cutaneous lupus might notice red, scaly patches on sun-exposed areas like the face, neck, and arms. These skin symptoms can be a clue that lupus is present, even if internal organs aren't affected. In some cases, cutaneous lupus exists on its own, without developing into systemic lupus, but in others, it can be an early sign of something more widespread.

Another type is drug-induced lupus, which, as the name suggests, is triggered by certain medications. The symptoms can look a lot like systemic lupus, with joint pain, fever, and rashes, but the key difference is that drug-induced lupus usually goes away once the triggering medication is stopped. It's a temporary and reversible form of lupus, which is reassuring for many people who develop it. There's also neonatal lupus, which is incredibly rare and affects newborn babies. In these cases, certain autoantibodies from the mother cross into the baby's bloodstream, causing a temporary lupus-like illness at birth. Most babies recover fully within a few months, and long-term issues are rare, but it's a reminder of how complex lupus can be — sometimes even affecting people before they're born.

One of the biggest challenges with lupus, especially for patients and families, is sorting out the myths from the facts. A common myth is that lupus is contagious, which it absolutely isn't. You can't catch lupus from someone else, not through touch, not through the air, not through anything. It's not an infection — it's your own immune system malfunctioning. Another misunderstanding is that lupus is a type of cancer. It's true that both diseases involve the immune system, but lupus has nothing to do with cancer. It doesn't spread like cancer, and it doesn't grow like cancer. However, because some treatments for lupus involve medications that also happen to be used in cancer, it's easy to see where that confusion comes from. Another widespread myth is that lupus always causes a butterfly rash across the face. While this rash is one of the more recognizable signs of lupus, not everyone gets it, and plenty of people with lupus never develop any visible skin symptoms at all. In fact, part of what makes lupus so tricky is that it can look completely different from one person to the next. For some, it's mainly joint pain and crushing fatigue. For others, it's kidney issues picked up in routine blood work. There's no single blueprint for lupus, which is why no two journeys with the disease are exactly alike.

There's also a dangerous myth that lupus isn't a serious disease. Because symptoms can come and go, and because many people with lupus look completely fine on the outside, some people assume it's not that big a deal. But lupus can be very serious, even life-threatening in some cases, especially if vital organs like the kidneys or heart are involved. On the other hand, there's also the myth that everyone with lupus is destined for severe disease and disability. The truth, as always, lies somewhere in the middle. With modern treatments and good care, many people with lupus lead long, active lives, even if the path is sometimes challenging.

Understanding lupus means making peace with uncertainty. It's a shape-shifter of a disease, capable of changing over time, surprising both patients and doctors. But it's not unbeatable, and knowledge really is power. The more you understand about what's happening inside your body, the better you can advocate for yourself, work with your doctors, and take the small, everyday steps that help protect your health. Lupus is complex, but your ability to understand it doesn't have to be. Every question you ask, every piece of knowledge you gain, puts you back in control — and that's one of the most powerful tools you can have.

CHAPTER 2: WHAT CAUSES LUPUS?

Lupus is one of those conditions that makes people ask, why me? It's a fair question, and it's one doctors and researchers have been trying to answer for decades. Unfortunately, there's no simple answer — not yet, anyway. What we do know is that lupus doesn't come from a single cause. There's no single virus, no one bad gene, no particular food or lifestyle choice that sets it off. Instead, lupus seems to be the result of a complicated mix of factors — some you're born with and some you're exposed to throughout your life. Understanding what scientists know so far can help make sense of why lupus happens, even if we don't have every piece of the puzzle yet.

At the center of lupus is your immune system, which is supposed to be your body's defense system. Normally, the immune system's job is to protect you from harmful invaders like bacteria, viruses, and other germs. It's a highly trained, incredibly smart system that can tell the difference between friend and foe — between your own healthy tissues and something that doesn't belong. In lupus, that system loses its ability to make that distinction. Instead of only attacking invaders, it mistakenly attacks your own cells, tissues, and organs. This "friendly fire" is what leads to the symptoms of lupus, whether it's joint pain, skin rashes, or more serious complications in the kidneys or heart. The technical term for this is autoimmunity, meaning the immune system is turning against itself.

So why does the immune system go rogue in some people and not others? That's where genetics come in. Having a certain combination of genes can make you more likely to develop lupus. But — and this is very important — having those genes doesn't mean you're guaranteed to get lupus. It's more like having the ingredients for a recipe; whether or not the final dish ever gets made depends on many other factors. Scientists have identified dozens of genes that are linked to lupus, many of which are involved in how the immune system functions. But genes alone don't tell the whole story. In fact, most people with a family history of lupus never develop the disease themselves, and many people diagnosed with lupus don't have anyone else in their family with it. Genetics creates the background risk, but something else has to trigger the disease into action.

That's where environmental triggers come in. These are things you encounter in the world around you that might "wake up" lupus if you already have the genetic tendency. One well-known trigger is infections. Certain viral infections, particularly Epstein-Barr virus (the virus that causes mononucleosis, or "mono"), have been linked to lupus in some studies. The theory is that these infections might confuse the immune system, training it to react too aggressively, which can eventually lead to autoimmune diseases like lupus in people who are already genetically vulnerable.

Sunlight is another common trigger, especially for people with cutaneous lupus or those who develop the classic butterfly rash. In people with lupus, exposure to ultraviolet (UV) light can cause the immune system to flare up, leading to skin rashes and even triggering full-body flares. It doesn't mean you have to live in the dark, but it does mean that sun protection becomes an important part of managing lupus.

Certain medications can also trigger lupus-like symptoms in some people. This type of lupus, called drug-induced lupus, is temporary and usually goes away once the medication is stopped. Not everyone who takes these medications will develop lupus symptoms — it depends on your individual immune system makeup. Common culprits include some blood pressure medications, certain anti-seizure drugs, and even some antibiotics.

Stress, both physical and emotional, is another potential trigger. Severe stress — from an accident, major surgery, or intense personal trauma — can sometimes be the tipping point that brings lupus symptoms to the surface for the first time. While stress doesn't cause lupus on its own, it can push an already overactive immune system into overdrive, leading to symptoms.

All of these triggers — infections, sunlight,

medications, and stress — are important, but they only trigger lupus in people who already have the underlying genetic risk. If you don't have the genetic tendency, you could go through all of these experiences and never develop lupus. It's this combination of genetics and environment — what some doctors call the perfect storm — that sets the stage for lupus to develop.

When it comes to who's at risk, there are some clear patterns. Gender is one of the strongest risk factors. About 9 out of 10 lupus patients are women, especially women of childbearing age, which means hormones likely play a role too. Estrogen, the primary female hormone, seems to interact with the immune system in ways that make autoimmunity more likely, although researchers are still working to fully understand how.

Age matters too. Lupus can develop at any age, but most people are diagnosed between the ages of 15 and 45 — the years when estrogen levels are highest. That doesn't mean older adults and children can't get lupus, but it's much less common in those age groups.

Ethnicity is another important piece of the risk puzzle. Lupus is more common, and often more severe, in people of African, Hispanic, Asian, and Native American descent compared to people of European descent. Researchers think this might be due to a combination of genetic factors and differences in environmental exposures, healthcare access, and social stressors. It's not just about who gets lupus — it's also about how severe it is and how well it responds to treatment.

Lupus doesn't have a single cause, and that can feel frustrating when you just want a clear explanation. But understanding this mix of genes, environment, gender, age, and ethnicity can help put your own lupus story into context. It's not something you caused. It's not something you could have prevented. It's the result of factors largely beyond your control — and knowing that can help you move forward with less guilt and more focus on what you can do to manage your health today.

Even though we don't yet know every trigger or every gene involved, researchers are making progress every year. By participating in research studies, sharing your story, and staying informed, you're not only helping yourself — you're helping doctors and scientists understand lupus better, so that future generations might have clearer answers and, hopefully, better treatments or even a cure. In the meantime, understanding the science — even in a simplified form — gives you power. It gives you language to explain what's happening to your body and helps you push back against blame, stigma, or the myth that you did something wrong. Lupus is complex, but you don't have to be a scientist to understand it, and every piece of knowledge you gain helps you take better care of yourself — and that's something to feel good about.

CHAPTER 3: EARLY SYMPTOMS

Lupus is often called the great imitator because its early symptoms can look like so many other illnesses. It doesn't come with a single clear signal, no flashing sign that says "this is lupus." Instead, it starts with a handful of symptoms that could mean almost anything — or nothing at all. That's part of what makes it so frustrating, both for patients and for doctors trying to figure out what's going on. One of the earliest and most common symptoms is fatigue, and this isn't the ordinary tiredness everyone feels after a long day or a bad night's sleep. This is a deep, bone-heavy exhaustion that doesn't go away with rest. People often describe it as feeling like they're moving through wet cement, where even simple tasks like taking a shower or making breakfast feel overwhelming. Fatigue can be one of the very first signs of lupus, sometimes appearing months or even years before other symptoms, but because fatigue is so common — caused by stress, poor sleep, low iron, thyroid problems, or even just life — it's rarely recognized as a red flag on its own.

Another common early symptom is joint pain, which can feel a lot like the aches of overuse or mild arthritis. But lupus joint pain often has some telltale features. It tends to be symmetrical, meaning it affects both sides of the body — both hands, both wrists, both knees — rather than just one. It's often worse in the morning and improves as you move around, though some people find it sticks with them all day. The joints might feel stiff, tender, or slightly swollen, but unlike in conditions like rheumatoid arthritis, lupus joint damage is often less severe. That said, the pain itself can be just as disruptive, making it hard to grip things, climb stairs, or go about daily life without discomfort.

Skin rashes can also show up early, especially after time in the sun. The classic lupus rash is the butterfly rash — a red or pink rash that stretches across the cheeks and nose like a pair of wings. It's one of the more recognizable lupus signs, but not everyone gets it. Some people develop red, scaly patches on their arms, neck, or chest, often in areas exposed to sunlight. Others notice sudden sensitivity to the sun itself — skin that used to tolerate the sun just fine suddenly reacts with redness or burning after only brief exposure. For some, skin changes are the very first clue that something's wrong, long before they feel sick in any other way.

Fever is another piece of the early lupus puzzle, though it's a tricky one. Many people with early lupus have unexplained low-grade fevers — not high enough to seem like a clear infection, but enough to feel off. These fevers tend to come and go, sometimes lasting a few hours, sometimes a few days, without any clear reason. They often arrive with fatigue and body aches, creating a flu-like feeling that never quite turns into a full-blown illness. Like fatigue, a low-grade fever is easy to brush off, especially if it resolves on its own, but in the context of other symptoms, it can be an important clue.

Alongside these common signs, lupus has a collection of unusual symptoms that can confuse even experienced doctors. Some people develop chest pain, especially when taking a deep breath. This can be a sign of pleurisy, an inflammation of the lining around the lungs, which is sometimes the first clear sign of lupus. Others develop mouth or nose ulcers, often painless but stubborn, appearing again and again even when you feel otherwise fine. Some people notice their fingers turn blue or white in the cold, a condition called Raynaud's phenomenon, caused by overreactive blood vessels. And then there are the symptoms that seem to have nothing to do with each other — random hair loss, headaches, dry eyes, unexplained weight loss, even memory lapses or trouble finding words. These scattered signs, when taken individually, rarely scream lupus, which is why the disease so often hides in plain sight, blending into other explanations until someone connects the dots.

One of the most important things to understand about lupus — and something that makes those early symptoms even harder to interpret — is that it doesn't follow a straight line. It's a disease of flares and remission, meaning symptoms come and go. A week of overwhelming fatigue might be followed by a month where you feel mostly normal. Joint pain might flare up after a stressful event and then disappear again. Skin rashes might come and go with changes in weather, stress, or sun exposure. This unpredictable, waxing and waning nature is part of what makes lupus so hard to catch early, especially when the first symptoms are mild or vague.

This stop-and-start pattern also plays tricks on your mind. You might start to think you imagined how bad you felt last week because today you feel fine. Friends, family, even doctors might assume that if you look good today, the problem must be gone. But that's the nature of lupus — it ebbs and flows, sometimes dramatically, sometimes quietly, and the intensity can change over time. What starts as mild joint pain might, years later, turn into kidney problems or chest pain. Or you might have one isolated flare and then go years without any trouble. No two lupus journeys are exactly alike, which is why learning to listen to your body — and trusting what it's telling you, even if no one else can see it — is such an important part of living with lupus.

In those early stages, the most important thing you can do is pay attention. Keep track of symptoms, even if they seem unrelated or unimportant. Write down how you feel after a day in the sun or after a stressful week. Notice patterns — do certain foods, weather changes, or activities make symptoms worse? Lupus is rarely diagnosed based on one symptom alone. It's the whole picture — the combination of symptoms over time, the waxing and waning pattern, the way symptoms cluster together — that eventually helps doctors make sense of what's happening. But the earliest clues come from you, from the changes you notice and the story only your body can tell. Listening to your body — and believing what it's saying — is one of the most valuable tools you have, even when lupus is still a mystery.

CHAPTER 4: HOW IS LUPUS DIAGNOSED?

Lupus is not the kind of disease that announces itself clearly. It doesn't show up on a single blood test or leave one unmistakable fingerprint that doctors can immediately recognize. Instead, diagnosing lupus is a slow process of gathering clues, putting together pieces of a puzzle that doesn't always come with a clear picture on the box. In many cases, it's not just about what tests show, but also about how symptoms evolve over time and how closely doctors are paying attention to those changes. That's why the process of diagnosing lupus often begins with something much simpler than a fancy test — it starts with a conversation. Your doctor will want to hear your story — when your symptoms started, how they've changed, what makes them better or worse, and whether anyone in your family has ever had anything like this. Because lupus tends to touch so many different parts of the body, your answers might span everything from joint pain to weird skin rashes to episodes of unexplained fatigue and fevers. Even things that might not seem connected — like mouth ulcers or fingers turning blue in the cold — could turn out to be important clues. This is why taking the time to paint a full picture for your doctor matters. Every symptom is a brushstroke, and the clearer the picture, the easier it becomes to see whether lupus might be the underlying cause.

After gathering your history, the doctor will perform a physical exam, looking for some of the outward signs of lupus. They might check your skin for rashes, especially in areas exposed to the sun. They'll gently press on your joints, looking for swelling, warmth, or tenderness. They might listen to your heart and lungs, check for swollen lymph nodes, and look at your hands and nails for signs of Raynaud's phenomenon or unusual capillary changes. None of these findings are diagnostic on their own, but together, they help build a case for or against lupus.

Once the story and the physical exam start to raise suspicion, the next step is usually a set of blood tests. One of the most important is called the ANA test, short for antinuclear antibody. This test looks for antibodies — immune system proteins — that mistakenly target parts of your own cells, particularly the nucleus, which is the control center of every cell. A positive ANA doesn't mean you definitely have lupus, but it's a strong clue, especially if your symptoms match. The vast majority of people with lupus have a positive ANA, but many healthy people can also have a positive ANA, so it's not a yes-or-no test. Instead, it's one piece of the puzzle. If the ANA is positive, your doctor will likely order more specific antibody tests, like anti-dsDNA and anti-

Smith antibodies, which are much more closely linked to lupus. Anti-dsDNA, in particular, is often associated with lupus nephritis, a type of kidney involvement, so doctors take it seriously. Other blood markers, like complement levels, may also be checked. Complement proteins are part of the immune system's defense system, and in lupus, low complement levels can indicate that your immune system is actively attacking tissues. Other tests might look for antiphospholipid antibodies, which can increase the risk of blood clots, another potential complication of lupus.

In addition to blood tests, urine tests are often part of the diagnostic process, especially if there's any concern about lupus affecting your kidneys. Your doctor might check for protein or blood in your urine, which can be early signs of lupus nephritis. Because the kidneys don't always cause noticeable symptoms until damage is already underway, these urine tests are an important part of catching kidney involvement as early as possible.

Imaging tests, like chest X-rays or echocardiograms, might also be ordered if you're having symptoms like chest pain or shortness of breath, to check for inflammation around the lungs or heart. Imaging can't diagnose lupus directly, but it can help doctors understand whether inflammation is affecting certain organs, which might point to lupus as a possible cause.

Despite all these tests, diagnosing lupus is rarely quick or straightforward. Part of the reason is that lupus doesn't always show itself fully right away. You might show up at the doctor's office with joint pain, but no rash. Or maybe you have fatigue and a positive ANA, but no kidney problems or fevers. Because lupus is so unpredictable, some people only meet the official diagnostic criteria after months or even years of accumulating symptoms. Doctors often wait and watch, repeating tests over time, to see whether a clearer pattern emerges. This process can be incredibly frustrating for patients, especially when they feel sick but don't have a name for what's happening to them. But it's not that doctors aren't taking your symptoms seriously — it's that lupus itself can be a slow reveal, unfolding in pieces rather than all at once.

Another complication is that lupus mimics so many other conditions. It's not the only disease that can cause joint pain, fatigue, fevers, and rashes, so part of the diagnostic process involves ruling out other possibilities. Conditions like rheumatoid arthritis, fibromyalgia, Sjögren's syndrome, and even some chronic infections can look a lot like lupus at first. Viral illnesses, especially ones like Epstein-Barr virus, can also cause temporary immune system changes that might mimic lupus, including a positive ANA. In some cases, doctors have to follow patients over time to see which pattern develops — does it resolve on its own, or does it gradually evolve into something that fits the criteria for lupus?

This is why lupus is often called a diagnosis of exclusion — meaning doctors have to rule out many other diseases before they feel confident that lupus is the right explanation. There's no single "lupus test" that gives a yes or no answer. Instead, it's the combination of symptoms, physical findings, blood and urine markers, and sometimes imaging results — all gathered over time — that eventually makes the diagnosis clear.

Even though the process can feel long and uncertain, it's important to stick with it. Lupus is much easier to manage when it's caught early, before it has a chance to cause serious organ damage. The sooner you have a diagnosis, the sooner you and your doctors can start working together on a treatment plan — one that not only controls symptoms but also protects your long-term health. And even if it takes time to get a clear diagnosis, every test, every conversation, every new clue brings you one step closer to understanding what's happening in your body — and that knowledge is powerful.

CHAPTER 5: UNDERSTANDING FLARES AND REMISSION

Lupus doesn't follow a straight road, and it certainly doesn't follow a schedule. Instead, it moves in waves — periods where symptoms worsen, called flares, followed by stretches where you feel better, known as remission. These ups and downs are part of the unpredictable rhythm of lupus, and learning to recognize and navigate them is one of the most important parts of living with the disease. For many people, the word flare sounds dramatic, like something sudden and explosive. But lupus flares can be subtle, building slowly over days or even weeks, while others hit like a truck out of nowhere. A flare simply means that the disease has become more active — the immune system, which might have been quiet for a while, is suddenly overreacting again, attacking healthy tissues and causing new or worsening symptoms. Flares are different for everyone, and no two are exactly alike, even in the same person. One flare might focus on your joints, while the next might bring crushing fatigue or skin rashes. The key is that something changes — a symptom you thought was under control suddenly gets worse, or new problems appear that weren't there before.

One of the hardest parts about flares is

understanding what triggers them. Sometimes the cause is clear — an infection, a period of intense stress, too much sun exposure — but other times, there's no obvious explanation at all. That's part of what makes lupus so frustrating. Still, there are some common triggers that show up again and again in people with lupus, and understanding them can help you reduce your risk or catch a flare early. Infections, even minor ones like a cold or a stomach bug, can spark a flare by revving up your immune system, which is already too active. Sunlight, particularly ultraviolet (UV) light, is another major trigger, especially for those with skin involvement. Even brief sun exposure can set off rashes and joint pain, and sometimes it triggers full-body symptoms. Stress, whether physical (like surgery or injury) or emotional (like a major life event), can also push your immune system into overdrive. Hormonal shifts, like pregnancy, menopause, or even changes in birth control, can sometimes set off flares in some people. Even certain medications, particularly antibiotics, blood pressure drugs, and hormone therapies, have been known to worsen lupus symptoms in susceptible people.

One of the most useful skills you can develop with lupus is learning to recognize the early signs that a flare might be starting. Often, the body sends subtle warnings before symptoms fully explode, and catching these signals early can sometimes help you take steps to soften or even prevent a full-blown flare. Some people notice a return of deep fatigue — that all-encompassing exhaustion that feels like moving through quicksand. Others get a low-grade fever, the kind that doesn't seem serious on its own but feels like a warning light. Joint pain and stiffness that creeps back into your hands or knees can also be a clue, even if the pain is milder than in past flares. For those with skin involvement, a new rash or sudden sun sensitivity can be an early red flag. Some people feel it in their mood — a sense of fogginess, irritability, or just knowing something isn't right. These early signs aren't always obvious, and it can take time to learn your own patterns, but the more you tune into your body, the better you'll get at spotting trouble before it fully arrives.

Once a flare starts, the next big question is always: how long will this last? The frustrating truth is that there's no single answer. Some flares are brief, lasting only a few days or a week. Others drag on for weeks or even months, requiring changes in treatment or higher doses of medications like steroids to bring them under control. There's no set timeline, and even within the same person, flare durations can vary widely. What's important to know is that flares do end, even if it doesn't feel like it in the middle of one. With the right treatment and self-care, the immune system can be coaxed back into a quieter state, even if it takes some time to get there. Understanding that flares are temporary, even if they're disruptive, can help you hold onto hope when things feel overwhelming.

The other side of the coin — and something many people with lupus find equally confusing — is remission. In some diseases, remission means the illness is completely gone, with no symptoms and no need for treatment. But in lupus, remission is more complicated. For some, remission might mean that symptoms are minimal or entirely absent, but they still need to stay on medications to keep the disease under control. This is called treatment-controlled remission, and it's actually quite common. For others, remission might mean they feel well without medication, which is called drug-free remission, but this is much rarer in lupus. Even in remission, many people still experience some mild symptoms, like fatigue or occasional joint pain, but if their bloodwork is stable and their organs are healthy, doctors might still consider them to be in a form of remission.

Remission can also be fragile. It's not a permanent state, and many people with lupus cycle in and out of remission over the years. The goal isn't necessarily to achieve a perfect, symptom-free life forever — though that's certainly possible for some — but rather to minimize flares, protect your organs, and maintain the best quality of life you can. Even if your lupus never fully "goes away," learning to manage it so that flares are rare, mild, and short is still a major victory. The longer you live with lupus, the more you'll come to understand your own rhythm — what triggers you, what helps you recover, and what signals to watch for. You'll become an expert in your own body, able to spot the whispers of a flare before they turn into a roar, and able to make choices — about rest, medications, sun exposure, and stress management — that help keep your lupus as quiet as possible.

Flares and remission are the natural ebb and flow of lupus. They can feel unpredictable, even unfair at times, but they're also not random. With each flare you go through, you gain more knowledge about how lupus behaves in your body, and that knowledge can be your most powerful tool in shaping what comes next. No one can predict exactly when a flare will hit or how long it will last, but by understanding what a flare is, what triggers it, and how to listen to your body's early signals, you can turn that unpredictability into something you understand and respond to — not something you have to fear. Lupus may have its own rhythm, but with time and attention, you can learn to dance with it, rather than constantly feel knocked off your feet.

CHAPTER 6: MEDICATIONS

When it comes to managing lupus, medications are not just optional tools — they're essential lifelines. They help calm an overactive immune system, protect vital organs, and ease the symptoms that can make daily life difficult. But because lupus can affect so many parts of the body, there's no single medication that works for everyone, and most people with lupus end up needing a combination of medications to keep their disease under control. The goal is never to pile on as many drugs as possible — it's to find the right balance between keeping the immune system quiet and minimizing side effects. That balance is different for everyone, and it often changes over time, depending on how active your lupus is and which parts of your body are affected.

At the center of almost every lupus treatment plan is a medication called hydroxychloroquine, sometimes known by the brand name Plaquenil. It's one of the oldest and most trusted drugs for lupus, and it's considered a cornerstone of treatment. Hydroxychloroquine isn't a fast-acting medication — it can take several months to fully kick in — but once it does, it's like a safety net for your immune system, gently calming the overreaction that drives lupus flares. It also has a protective effect, lowering the risk of serious organ damage over the long term.

Even people whose lupus is relatively mild are often kept on hydroxychloroquine for years, sometimes for life, because of its disease-modifying benefits. It's one of the safest lupus medications, but it does require regular eye exams, since in very rare cases, it can affect the retina. These checks are usually once a year, and the vast majority of people take hydroxychloroquine for decades without any eye problems at all.

While hydroxychloroquine works quietly in the background, steroids often play a more dramatic role in managing lupus flares. These are not the steroids used by bodybuilders — they're corticosteroids, like prednisone, which act as powerful anti-inflammatory drugs. In the middle of a severe flare, when the immune system is attacking joints, skin, kidneys, or even the heart or lungs, steroids can work within hours to rapidly bring inflammation under control. They're fast, they're effective, and sometimes they're the only thing standing between a person and serious organ damage. But they come with a price, especially when used long-term. High doses or prolonged courses of steroids can cause weight gain, insomnia, mood changes, high blood sugar, high blood pressure, osteoporosis, and increased infection risk. That's why doctors work so hard to minimize steroid use — using them just long enough to bring flares under control, then slowly tapering down to the lowest possible dose or stopping them altogether if the disease allows. Steroids can be life-saving, but they're also a double-edged sword, requiring careful monitoring and a willingness to balance short-term control with long-term health.

For people whose lupus can't be managed with hydroxychloroquine and occasional steroids alone — especially those with serious organ involvement — doctors often add a class of drugs called immunosuppressants. These medications — including methotrexate, mycophenolate mofetil (CellCept), and azathioprine (Imuran) — work by dampening the immune system's overactivity. They're often described as immune system brakes, helping prevent flares by slowing down the immune response before it can cause damage. Each of these medications has its own strengths and considerations. Methotrexate is often used for joint and skin symptoms, while mycophenolate is more commonly used for lupus nephritis, which affects the kidneys. Azathioprine can be used for a variety of lupus manifestations, and it's sometimes preferred for people planning pregnancy because it's safer in pregnancy than some other immunosuppressants. These medications work well for many people, but because they suppress the immune system, they can increase the risk of infections, so regular blood tests are essential to make sure your immune system isn't being suppressed too much.

In recent years, a newer class of medications

called biologics has started to play a bigger role in lupus treatment. These are highly targeted therapies designed to block specific parts of the immune system that drive lupus. The first biologic approved specifically for lupus was belimumab (Benlysta), which works by blocking a protein called BLyS, which helps lupus B cells (the cells that make antibodies) survive longer than they should. By removing excess BLyS, belimumab can reduce disease activity and cut down on flares in some people, especially those with milder forms of lupus who still struggle with frequent symptoms despite traditional medications. More recently, anifrolumab (Saphnelo) was approved. It works by blocking interferon, a key inflammatory protein involved in lupus. Anifrolumab seems to work particularly well for skin and joint symptoms, and it's given as an infusion, meaning it's delivered directly into a vein. Biologics aren't for everyone, and they tend to be used when more traditional medications haven't worked well enough. They're expensive, but they represent a new wave of targeted treatment, giving hope to people whose lupus has been hard to control.

Whatever combination of medications you're on, managing side effects becomes a key part of living with lupus. No medication is completely free of side effects, and balancing symptom control with safety is always the goal. Some side effects are short-term and manageable, like mild nausea or fatigue when starting a new drug. Others, like infection risk, bone thinning, or liver problems, need ongoing monitoring with regular blood tests and check-ups. It's important to report any new symptoms to your doctor, even if they seem unrelated to lupus. Sometimes, side effects can be reduced by adjusting the dose, changing the timing of medications, or adding medications to protect against complications, like calcium and vitamin D for bone health. Medications can feel like a double-edged sword, but when used carefully and monitored closely, they are often the key to keeping lupus under control while protecting your long-term health.

The importance of regular follow-ups cannot be overstated. Lupus is not a set-it-and-forget-it disease, and your treatment needs will evolve over time. What works during a flare may not be needed during remission, and new symptoms can require changes to your medication plan. Seeing your doctor regularly — even when you're feeling well — helps catch early signs of trouble before they become serious. These visits are a chance to check your bloodwork, monitor for side effects, and make sure your medications are still the right fit for your current symptoms. It's also an opportunity to ask questions, discuss new research, and talk about how lupus is affecting your life beyond the lab results. Your medications are important, but so is your voice — the more you share about how you're feeling, the better your doctor can tailor your treatment to match your real life, not just your test results.

Lupus medications can feel overwhelming, especially when you're first diagnosed. It's not uncommon to feel like you're suddenly a walking pharmacy, with pills, infusions, and check-ups becoming part of your new normal. But over time, you'll come to understand which medications help you the most, which side effects are worth tolerating, and which are not. You'll become an expert in your own version of lupus, and that expertise — combined with the right medications and a strong partnership with your healthcare team — will help you stay in control, even when lupus itself tries to take the wheel. Medications aren't the whole story, but they are a powerful set of tools, and knowing how to use them wisely is one of the most important steps in building a life where lupus doesn't define you.

CHAPTER 7: MONITORING YOUR HEALTH

Living with lupus isn't just about managing symptoms when they appear — it's about staying one step ahead of the disease, even when you're feeling well. Because lupus has the potential to affect almost every part of your body, regular checkups and routine monitoring tests become an essential part of your care. These aren't just random blood draws or box-ticking exercises; they are windows into how your immune system is behaving, how your organs are holding up, and how well your medications are protecting you. Lupus is often quiet, especially in its early stages, and damage to vital organs like the kidneys, heart, and bones can build up silently before any obvious symptoms appear. That's why even when you feel perfectly fine, these regular tests and checkups are some of the most important tools for protecting your long-term health.

At the core of your monitoring routine are blood and urine tests, which give doctors a direct look at how active your lupus is and whether your treatment plan is keeping the disease in check. Blood tests can check for inflammation markers, like ESR (erythrocyte sedimentation rate) and CRP (C-reactive protein), which rise when the immune system is flaring up. Other tests check your complete blood count (CBC), looking for signs of anemia, low white blood cells, or low platelets — all of which can be affected by lupus itself or by the medications used to treat it. Your doctor will also keep an eye on your kidney function, since lupus nephritis — inflammation in the kidneys — is one of the most serious potential complications of lupus. This means regular checks of creatinine and glomerular filtration rate (GFR) to see how well your kidneys are filtering waste. Urine tests are equally important, especially if your lupus has ever affected your kidneys. Urine protein levels and urine sediment can reveal early signs of kidney trouble long before you feel anything. Even when you feel healthy, these tests help your doctor catch subtle signs of a lupus flare before it turns into something more serious.

Another area that requires attention, especially if you've been on steroids for any length of time, is your bone health. Corticosteroids like prednisone are powerful tools for controlling inflammation, but they come with a long list of potential side effects — and bone thinning, or osteoporosis, is one of the most concerning. Even people with lupus who haven't used steroids long-term can be at risk for weaker bones, partly because lupus itself can contribute to inflammation in the bones and joints. That's why bone density scans — also known as DEXA scans — are recommended for many people with lupus. These painless, non-invasive scans measure the strength of your bones and can help identify early signs of bone thinning, long before fractures become a risk. If your bones are starting to weaken, your doctor can recommend calcium and vitamin D supplements, weight-bearing exercise, or even medications to help protect your bones before real damage occurs.

If hydroxychloroquine is part of your lupus treatment plan — and for most people, it is — regular eye exams are also essential. Although hydroxychloroquine is generally considered one of the safest long-term lupus medications, it does carry a small risk of damage to the retina, the part of your eye responsible for detailed vision. This risk is extremely low in the first few years of treatment, but it increases the longer you're on the medication, especially after five years or more. That's why annual retinal screenings with an ophthalmologist who understands lupus are so important. These eye exams involve not just a standard vision check, but also specialized imaging to look for very early signs of retinal changes — changes you wouldn't notice yourself until they're more advanced. If caught early, these changes are usually reversible, and in most cases, the benefits of staying on hydroxychloroquine far outweigh the small risk to your vision. But regular screening ensures that if any problems do develop, they can be caught early and managed before they become serious.

Because lupus can also affect your heart and blood vessels, monitoring your cardiovascular health is another key piece of the puzzle. People with lupus have a higher risk of developing atherosclerosis, or hardening of the arteries, even at younger ages. This is partly due to chronic inflammation, which can damage blood vessels over time, and partly due to the side effects of some lupus medications, like steroids, which can increase cholesterol and blood pressure. That's why your doctor will regularly check your cholesterol levels, blood pressure, and sometimes recommend echocardiograms or other imaging to look at your heart if you're experiencing chest pain, shortness of breath, or other symptoms that might suggest inflammation in the heart or the lining around it. Taking steps to keep your heart healthy, like not smoking, eating a balanced diet, and getting regular exercise, becomes especially important when you have lupus.

Kidney health also needs ongoing attention, especially if you've ever had lupus nephritis. Even if your kidneys are currently stable, regular blood and urine tests are essential to catch the earliest signs of trouble. Lupus nephritis doesn't always cause noticeable symptoms until significant damage has already been done, so monitoring kidney function — and making adjustments to your medications if needed — is a key part of protecting your long-term health. If you have a history of kidney involvement, your nephrologist might also recommend kidney ultrasounds or biopsies at certain points to directly assess how your kidneys are holding up.

Vaccinations are another area where lupus care requires a bit of extra attention. Because many lupus medications suppress your immune system, certain vaccines — particularly live vaccines, like the measles-mumps-rubella (MMR) vaccine or the shingles vaccine — are usually off-limits while you're on immunosuppressants. But that doesn't mean vaccines are unimportant. In fact, staying up to date on recommended vaccines is one of the best ways to protect yourself from infections, which can be serious or even life-threatening when you have lupus. Annual flu shots, pneumonia vaccines, and COVID-19 vaccines are especially important, since infections can not only make you very sick, but also trigger lupus flares. If you're unsure which vaccines are safe for you, your rheumatologist can help create a personalized vaccination plan that balances your need for protection against infection with the safety concerns related to your medications.

Staying on top of all these tests, checkups, and screenings can feel overwhelming at first, but over time, they become part of your rhythm — regular checkpoints that give you and your doctors the information you need to keep your lupus under control and catch problems early. They're not just about watching for flares; they're about protecting your future health, even when your lupus is quiet. Each blood test, each scan, each eye exam is another piece of information that helps you and your medical team make the best possible decisions about your care. It's easy to think of these checkups as something you do for your doctor, but they're really something you do for yourself — for your future, for your quality of life, for your peace of mind. In lupus, knowledge is power, and the more you know about how your body is doing, the more confident you can feel that you're staying ahead of the disease, not just reacting to it. Regular monitoring is not about expecting bad news — it's about making sure you're always in the best possible position to stay healthy, stay active, and stay in control, no matter what lupus throws your way.

CHAPTER 8: LUPUS AND YOUR ORGANS

Lupus is sometimes described as the disease with a thousand faces, and nowhere is that more true than in the way it affects the organs and systems throughout your body. It's a condition driven by an immune system that can't quite tell the difference between what's part of you and what's an enemy, so it turns its weapons inward, attacking your own tissues by mistake. Because your immune system reaches into every corner of your body — from your skin to your joints to your heart and brain — lupus has the potential to cause problems in almost any organ. No two people with lupus experience the exact same set of problems, and the pattern of organ involvement can change over time. Some people's lupus stays mostly on the surface, causing skin rashes and joint pain, while others develop deeper organ involvement affecting the kidneys, heart, or brain. Understanding the ways lupus can touch different parts of your body can make it easier to recognize symptoms when they appear and to appreciate why regular monitoring is so important, even if you feel fine.

The skin is one of the most visible places lupus can make itself known, and for some people, it's the first and most persistent sign of the disease.

Rashes are common, particularly in areas exposed to sunlight, like the face, neck, and arms. The most famous lupus rash is the butterfly rash, a red or pink rash that spreads across the cheeks and bridge of the nose. But lupus can also cause other types of skin issues — round, scaly patches known as discoid lupus, or more generalized rashes that mimic eczema or allergic reactions. The skin in lupus is often extra-sensitive to sunlight, and even a few minutes of unprotected sun exposure can trigger redness, burning, or the sudden appearance of a rash. This photosensitivity isn't just a nuisance — in some people, it can actually trigger whole-body flares, making sun protection an important part of managing the disease. Hair loss is another common issue, sometimes linked to the scalp itself being inflamed, and other times tied to the stress of a flare or the medications used to treat it. The good news is that lupus-related hair loss is often reversible, especially when the underlying inflammation is brought under control.

Joints and muscles are also frequent targets, with arthritis being one of the most common symptoms of lupus. Lupus arthritis usually affects the small joints — fingers, wrists, knees — and tends to be symmetrical, meaning it hits both sides of the body at the same time. The pain can range from mild stiffness to more severe swelling and tenderness, and it's often worse in the morning or after periods of rest. Unlike some other types of arthritis, like rheumatoid arthritis, lupus arthritis doesn't usually cause permanent joint damage, though it can certainly make daily tasks difficult during a flare. Muscle aches, or myalgia, are also common, sometimes from inflammation directly in the muscles and sometimes from the general strain lupus places on the body. Fatigue and inactivity during a flare can also contribute to muscle weakness, which is why gentle movement — even when you're not feeling your best — is often recommended to keep muscles from becoming deconditioned.

The kidneys are among the most important organs to monitor in lupus, because lupus nephritis, or inflammation of the kidneys, is one of the most serious complications the disease can cause. In the early stages, lupus nephritis is often completely silent, with no symptoms at all. That's why regular blood and urine tests are essential — they can catch subtle signs like protein or blood in the urine, or rising creatinine levels, long before you would feel anything. When lupus nephritis becomes more severe, it can cause symptoms like swelling in the legs and ankles, high blood pressure, or foamy urine. Lupus nephritis is treated aggressively, usually with immunosuppressants or biologic medications, because the goal is to protect as much kidney function as possible for as long as possible. Catching it early and staying on top of regular monitoring gives you the best chance of avoiding serious kidney damage down the road.

The heart and lungs are also vulnerable to inflammation from lupus, though the symptoms can be easy to overlook or blame on something else. Pericarditis, or inflammation of the lining around the heart, can cause sharp chest pain, especially when you lie down or take a deep breath. Pleuritis, or inflammation of the lining around the lungs, can cause a similar pleuritic chest pain, often made worse by deep breathing or coughing. Lupus can also increase your risk of atherosclerosis, the buildup of plaque inside your arteries, which can lead to heart attacks or strokes, sometimes at younger ages than expected. This risk isn't just due to lupus itself — steroids, often used to control flares, can also contribute to high blood pressure, high cholesterol, and weight gain, all of which increase heart risk. Regular heart checkups, blood pressure monitoring, and cholesterol checks are all part of keeping your heart and lungs safe, even when you're feeling well.

The brain and nervous system can also be affected by lupus, though this is one of the more mysterious and unpredictable areas of the disease. Some people experience cognitive dysfunction, often called lupus fog, which can make it hard to concentrate, remember things, or find the right words. This isn't just normal forgetfulness — it's a real neurological symptom of lupus, though it tends to come and go. Mood changes, like anxiety and depression, are also common in lupus, and they're not always just reactions to the stress of living with a chronic illness — they can be driven by underlying inflammation in the brain itself. In rare cases, lupus can cause more serious neurological symptoms, like seizures, strokes, or inflammation in the lining of the brain. Because these symptoms can mimic other conditions, they often require careful evaluation by both rheumatologists and neurologists, sometimes with additional tests like MRIs or spinal taps to sort out exactly what's happening.

Lupus can also affect the blood in a number of ways, some subtle and some potentially dangerous. Many people with lupus develop anemia, either because of chronic inflammation or as a side effect of medications. Low white blood cell counts are also common, though they're usually mild and don't cause symptoms. More concerning are problems with clotting, which can happen when lupus triggers antiphospholipid syndrome (APS) — a condition where the immune system produces antibodies that interfere with normal blood clotting. APS can increase the risk of blood clots in the legs (deep vein thrombosis), lungs (pulmonary embolism), and even the brain (stroke). Because of this risk, many people with lupus and APS are treated with blood thinners to prevent clots, especially if they've already had one clotting event.

The bottom line is that lupus doesn't just affect one part of your body — it can potentially touch every system, from your skin to your brain to your blood vessels. That's why whole-body care is so important, and why regular monitoring, even when you feel fine, is part of protecting your health over the long term. The good news is that no one develops every complication, and with the right medications, monitoring, and lifestyle adjustments, most people with lupus can lead full, active lives. The key is understanding how your own version of lupus behaves, so you can watch for early signs of trouble and work with your medical team to stay ahead of the disease. Lupus might have the potential to affect your whole body, but it doesn't have to define your life — with knowledge, vigilance, and the right care, you can stay in control, even when lupus tries to move the goalposts.

CHAPTER 9: LUPUS AND FATIGUE

Fatigue in lupus is not like ordinary tiredness. It's not the kind of tired you feel after a busy day, or even the exhaustion that comes with a bad cold or the flu. It's a deep, all-encompassing, bone-weary fatigue that seems to come out of nowhere and refuses to leave, no matter how much you rest. Fatigue in lupus is often called an invisible symptom, because there's no rash, no swollen joint, nothing you can point to that explains why you feel the way you do. Other people might look at you and assume you're fine, because on the outside, you may look exactly the same. But inside, it feels like you're dragging a heavy weight around with you everywhere you go. This disconnect — between how you feel and how others see you — can be one of the most frustrating parts of living with lupus-related fatigue, and it's also one of the hardest parts to explain to family, friends, or even doctors.

The causes of this kind of fatigue are complicated, and rarely boil down to just one thing. Sometimes, the disease itself is driving the exhaustion — especially if there's active inflammation somewhere in your body. Your immune system, which normally works quietly in the background, becomes overactive in lupus, and that overactivity uses up a lot of energy. Think of it like leaving all the lights on in your house 24 hours a day — your body is burning through its reserves just trying to keep up with the constant inflammation. This type of inflammatory fatigue can be especially intense during or just after a flare, when your immune system has been working overtime. Even once the inflammation settles down, the aftershocks can leave you feeling drained for weeks.

But there are also medical causes for fatigue in lupus that go beyond inflammation itself. Anemia — low red blood cell counts — is common in lupus, either because of chronic inflammation interfering with how your body produces blood cells, or because of side effects from medications. When you don't have enough red blood cells to carry oxygen efficiently, everything feels harder, and fatigue becomes a constant companion. Thyroid problems, which are more common in people with lupus, can also sap your energy, leaving you feeling sluggish and foggy no matter how much sleep you get. Sleep disorders, like sleep apnea or restless leg syndrome, can be quietly robbing you of restful sleep without you even realizing it. Medications themselves — especially steroids, some immunosuppressants, and even pain medications — can also contribute to daytime fatigue, either directly or by interfering with your ability to get deep, restorative sleep.

Alongside these medical contributors, there are also lifestyle factors that can quietly amplify your fatigue. Stress — whether from work, relationships, finances, or just the emotional burden of living with lupus — can be profoundly draining. Emotional stress and physical stress tap into the same energy reserves, so if you're constantly carrying the weight of worry, frustration, or uncertainty, your energy tank is going to feel perpetually low. Poor diet, dehydration, and lack of physical activity also play a role. When you're exhausted, the last thing you feel like doing is cooking a healthy meal or going for a walk, but over time, poor nutrition and deconditioning can worsen fatigue even further, creating a vicious cycle that's hard to break.

One of the most helpful strategies for managing lupus fatigue is learning how to conserve and protect your energy, treating it like the limited and precious resource it is. This doesn't mean giving up on your life — it means being strategic about where your energy goes. Think of your energy like money in a checking account — if you overspend on one activity, there's nothing left for the rest of the day. Many people with lupus find that pacing is key — alternating periods of activity with planned rest breaks, rather than trying to power through until they collapse. It can be helpful to prioritize tasks, focusing your energy on the things that matter most, and learning to delegate or let go of things that aren't essential. It's not about being lazy — it's about protecting your health so that you can show up fully for the things that truly matter.

Sometimes, energy conservation means getting

creative. If standing to cook dinner feels impossible, sit on a stool while you chop vegetables. If running errands wipes you out, group them together so you only have to go out once. If social events leave you drained, be upfront with friends and family about needing shorter visits or quieter activities. These kinds of adjustments might feel awkward at first, especially if you're used to pushing through no matter what, but over time they become second nature — a way to live smarter, not harder.

Good sleep hygiene is another essential piece of the puzzle. Fatigue isn't always caused by poor sleep, but restorative sleep — the kind that leaves you feeling recharged — is especially important when you have lupus. Creating a consistent bedtime routine, where you go to sleep and wake up at the same times each day, helps regulate your body's internal clock. Avoiding screens and bright light for at least an hour before bed gives your brain time to wind down. Keeping your bedroom cool, dark, and quiet sets the stage for better sleep. If pain or discomfort makes it hard to sleep, investing in a supportive mattress or pillows, or using gentle stretching or heat therapy before bed, can help. And if your mind races the moment your head hits the pillow — running through worries about your health, your to-do list, or the future — practicing relaxation techniques, like deep breathing or guided imagery, can help your brain learn to slow down.

If despite all these adjustments your fatigue

remains overwhelming, it's worth having an honest conversation with your doctor. Sometimes, tweaking your medications, treating an underlying issue like anemia or thyroid dysfunction, or adjusting your approach to exercise and nutrition can make a difference. Fatigue is such a common and frustrating symptom of lupus that it deserves attention, even if it's not as dramatic as a skin rash or joint swelling. It's not "just part of having lupus" — it's a real, treatable symptom, and you don't have to simply accept it.

The most important thing to remember is that lupus fatigue is real, even if others can't see it. You are not weak, lazy, or imagining things. Your body is working overtime, fighting battles you can't always feel directly, and that fight uses energy. Recognizing that fatigue is part of the disease — and not a personal failure — helps you approach it with more compassion for yourself and less guilt. Learning to manage your energy, ask for help when you need it, and make peace with the fact that some days will be harder than others is all part of living well with lupus. Fatigue might be invisible to the outside world, but you feel it — and your experience matters, even if no one else can see the battle you're fighting inside.

CHAPTER 10: NUTRITION AND LUPUS: WHAT TO EAT (AND AVOID)

When it comes to lupus, food is not a cure, but it's also far more than just fuel. What you eat can either support your body's healing processes or make inflammation worse, and while diet alone won't stop lupus in its tracks, the right foods — combined with medications and other treatments — can help reduce flare risk, support organ health, and improve your overall quality of life. For many people with lupus, food becomes part of their self-care toolkit, a way to nourish not just their bodies but also their sense of control in a life often shaped by unpredictability. There's no single "lupus diet", but researchers have begun to understand more about how certain foods interact with inflammation and immunity, and that growing knowledge can help guide your choices in the kitchen.

At the heart of a lupus-friendly diet is the idea of anti-inflammatory eating — choosing foods that naturally help calm inflammation rather than fan the flames. This doesn't mean rigid rules or cutting out entire food groups, but rather leaning heavily on whole, nutrient-dense foods that support your body's healing processes. Colorful fruits and vegetables are rich in antioxidants, which help neutralize the free radicals that can worsen inflammation in lupus. Berries, leafy greens, sweet potatoes, and bell peppers are just a few examples of foods that deliver both vitamins and protective plant compounds. Fatty fish, like salmon, mackerel, and sardines, are packed with omega-3 fatty acids, which have been shown to reduce inflammation and may even help with joint pain and stiffness in autoimmune diseases like lupus. If fish isn't your thing, you can also get omega-3s from walnuts, chia seeds, and flaxseeds, though the body has to work a little harder to convert these plant sources into the active forms your body uses.

Healthy fats in general play an important role, especially olive oil, which is a core ingredient in anti-inflammatory eating patterns like the Mediterranean diet. Olive oil contains compounds that act as natural anti-inflammatories — in fact, some of these compounds work on similar pathways to ibuprofen, though much more gently. Legumes, whole grains like quinoa and brown rice, and a variety of nuts and seeds all help provide fiber, vitamins, and healthy fats, while also helping to keep blood sugar stable, which may also play a role in controlling inflammation. High fiber intake also feeds the beneficial bacteria in your gut, which may be particularly important for people with lupus — more on that in a moment.

Just as some foods help calm inflammation, others have the potential to worsen it — and these are the foods that are best limited, though not necessarily forbidden altogether. Excess salt can contribute to high blood pressure, which is already a concern for people with lupus, particularly if the kidneys or heart are affected. Salt can also worsen water retention, which is common in people on steroids, leaving you feeling puffy and uncomfortable. Processed and packaged foods are often loaded with sodium, along with artificial additives and preservatives, many of which have been linked to gut inflammation and immune dysregulation. It doesn't mean you have to swear off all convenience foods, but reading labels and choosing lower-sodium, minimally processed options when possible can make a real difference.

Added sugars and refined carbohydrates — think white bread, sugary cereals, candy, and soda — are also worth minimizing, not just because they contribute to weight gain (which can compound joint pain and fatigue), but because they can trigger spikes in blood sugar that may promote inflammatory processes in the body. This doesn't mean you can't have a treat now and then, but making sweets an occasional indulgence rather than a daily staple can help support your overall inflammation levels. Alcohol is another area where moderation matters. For many people with lupus, a small glass of wine with dinner isn't a problem, but alcohol can interact with some medications, stress the liver, and contribute to poor sleep, which can all indirectly worsen lupus symptoms. If you have lupus nephritis or liver involvement, your doctor may recommend avoiding alcohol entirely.

The world of supplements can be confusing, especially for people with lupus, who are often bombarded with claims about miracle vitamins or herbs that supposedly "cure" autoimmune disease. The reality is more nuanced. There's some evidence that omega-3 supplements — especially if you don't eat much fish — may be beneficial for reducing inflammation. Vitamin D is also worth paying attention to, since people with lupus often avoid the sun (for good reason), which is the body's natural way of producing vitamin D. Low vitamin D levels have been linked to worse lupus symptoms, so your doctor may recommend supplementing if your levels are low. Calcium is important too, particularly if you're on steroids, which can weaken bones over time. Beyond these basics, the evidence for supplements gets murkier. Some people with lupus experiment with turmeric, which has natural anti-inflammatory properties, but the results are inconsistent, and high doses could potentially interfere with medications. Herbal supplements, especially those marketed as immune boosters, should be approached with caution, since stimulating the immune system could potentially worsen autoimmunity rather than help. As with anything, it's best to check with your doctor before adding any supplement to your routine, even if it's something marketed as "natural."

In recent years, researchers have started paying more attention to the gut, and its potential role in autoimmune diseases like lupus. The gut microbiome — the trillions of bacteria living in your intestines — plays a surprisingly large role in immune system regulation. In healthy people, the gut helps train the immune system, teaching it how to tell friendly bacteria from harmful invaders. But in people with autoimmune diseases, this training process may go awry, possibly triggered by imbalances in gut bacteria or leaky gut, where small particles leak from the intestines into the bloodstream, triggering immune responses. While the science is still emerging, it's possible that supporting gut health could help calm the overactive immune response in lupus. That's one more reason why a fiber-rich, plant-based diet — which feeds the good bacteria in your gut — might be beneficial. Probiotic foods, like yogurt, kefir, sauerkraut, and kimchi, can help add beneficial bacteria directly, though it's unclear whether probiotic supplements offer the same benefits. The gut-lupus connection isn't fully understood yet, but it's an exciting area of research — and one that highlights how much what you eat might shape how your immune system behaves.

Ultimately, nutrition with lupus isn't about perfection — it's about creating a pattern of eating that supports your body's healing, gives you energy, and reduces your risk of complications like heart disease, osteoporosis, and kidney damage. It's about finding foods you enjoy that also happen to nourish your body, rather than approaching food as a rigid set of rules. There's room for flexibility, treats, and celebrations — as long as the foundation is built on whole, nutrient-dense, anti-inflammatory foods. Every meal is an opportunity to nourish not just your body, but your sense of well-being, to remind yourself that you have some control, even in the face of an unpredictable disease. Food won't cure lupus — but it can become a powerful ally, helping you feel stronger, calmer, and more in charge of your health, one meal at a time.

CHAPTER 11: EXERCISE AND MOVEMENT

Exercise can feel like a complicated subject when you're living with lupus. On one hand, you've probably heard that staying active is good for you — it strengthens your muscles, supports your heart, boosts your mood, and helps with fatigue. But on the other hand, when your body hurts, your joints are stiff, and you're already exhausted, the idea of exercise can feel impossible. It's not just the physical challenge — there's often a mental block too, the fear that moving too much could trigger a flare or make your symptoms worse. The truth, as with most things in lupus, is all about balance. The right kinds of gentle, regular movement can actually help you feel better, both physically and emotionally, but it's also true that overdoing it or choosing the wrong type of exercise can make things worse. Learning how to find that sweet spot — enough movement to help, but not so much that it pushes your body into rebellion — is one of the most valuable skills you can develop.

The benefits of gentle exercise in lupus go far beyond just burning calories or building muscle. Regular movement helps keep your joints flexible, which can be especially important when stiffness is one of your daily challenges. It also helps reduce inflammation, in part by improving circulation and in part by calming stress hormones like cortisol, which can feed inflammation when they're constantly elevated. Exercise also supports bone health, which is particularly important if you've ever been on steroids, since these medications can weaken bones over time. Perhaps most importantly, regular movement can improve fatigue, not by pushing through it, but by gently increasing your stamina over time. It might sound counterintuitive — after all, if you're exhausted, why would movement help? But research shows that staying active, even in small ways, helps reduce the deep, chronic fatigue that so many people with lupus live with every day. Movement also boosts endorphins, the brain's feel-good chemicals, which can lift your mood, ease anxiety, and even help with the brain fog that sometimes comes with lupus.

The key, though, is to choose the right types of exercise — activities that are gentle on the joints, easy to modify, and flexible enough to adjust based on how you're feeling that day. Walking is one of the simplest and best options for most people with lupus. It's free, it doesn't require special equipment, and you can go at your own pace, whether that's a short stroll around your neighborhood or a longer walk on a day when you have more energy. Walking helps improve circulation, supports heart health, and gently works your muscles without putting too much stress on your joints. It's also easy to break into short chunks, which is helpful if your energy comes in bursts — you can do 5 or 10 minutes at a time and still get real benefits.

Swimming and water exercise are also fantastic choices, especially if you have joint pain or stiffness. Water supports your body weight, taking pressure off your joints, while still allowing you to move through a full range of motion. The gentle resistance of the water helps strengthen muscles without the pounding that comes with high-impact exercise. Many community pools offer aqua aerobics classes specifically designed for people with arthritis or chronic illness, where the movements are slow, gentle, and easily adaptable to your individual needs. Being in the water can also be soothing, especially if you deal with muscle tension or nerve pain.

For those who prefer a more mind-body approach, yoga and tai chi are wonderful options. Yoga helps improve flexibility, balance, and strength, while also incorporating deep breathing and relaxation techniques that can help with stress management. The key is to choose gentle forms of yoga, like hatha or restorative yoga, rather than fast-paced power yoga styles. Tai chi, a slow, flowing martial art, offers similar benefits — gentle movement combined with focused breathing and mindfulness. Both practices emphasize listening to your body, which is exactly the mindset you need to exercise safely with lupus.

One of the most important lessons in lupus-friendly movement is understanding that more isn't always better. The goal isn't to push through pain or exhaustion — it's to work with your body, not against it. If you're having a good day, it's tempting to go all out, cramming in as much activity as possible. But that kind of boom-and-bust cycle, where you overdo it on good days and crash for the next several days, is counterproductive. Instead, the key is to develop a gentle, consistent routine, even if that means starting with just a few minutes a day. Consistency is more important than intensity. Over time, your body will gradually adapt, and you may find that your stamina improves, your pain decreases, and your flares become less frequent — all without ever pushing yourself to the point of collapse.

If joint pain and stiffness are a barrier, there are ways to work around that too. Warm up gently before any activity, using heat packs on stiff joints if needed. Start with slow, range-of-motion exercises, simply moving your joints through their comfortable range to get the synovial fluid flowing and lubricate your joints. If a particular joint is flaring, you can modify movements to avoid stressing that area — for example, using a stationary bike instead of walking if your knees are inflamed. Splints or braces can provide extra support for weak or painful joints, especially during weight-bearing activities. And if pain does flare up during or after exercise, rest, ice, and gentle stretching can help settle things down again.

The most important thing to remember is that exercise with lupus isn't about performance — it's about function. It's not about running marathons, lifting heavy weights, or hitting specific fitness goals. It's about keeping your body as strong, mobile, and resilient as possible, so you can live your life with more comfort and confidence. On some days, movement might mean a slow walk around the block or a few gentle stretches in your living room. On other days, you might feel up to a longer session or a class. Both are wins. The goal is to create a flexible relationship with movement, one that can adapt to the ups and downs of lupus, giving you the freedom to move when you can and rest when you need to, without guilt or pressure.

In the end, movement is less about checking off boxes and more about reconnecting with your body, learning what feels good, what helps, and what your limits are — and respecting those limits. Movement can become a kind of self-care, a way to show your body compassion, even when it feels like lupus has turned it into the enemy. With patience, creativity, and flexibility, exercise can shift from something you fear to something you look forward to — a gift you give yourself, one gentle step, stretch, or breath at a time.

CHAPTER 12: MENTAL HEALTH MATTERS

Lupus isn't just a disease of the body — it touches your mind, your emotions, your sense of identity, and the way you see your future. From the moment you first hear the word lupus, life shifts in ways that are hard to explain unless you've lived it yourself. There's the shock, the confusion, the endless Googling that brings up worst-case scenarios you wish you hadn't seen. There's the weight of a chronic diagnosis, the realization that this isn't something you're going to get over, like a cold or a broken bone, but something that's going to be part of your life forever. Even if your symptoms are mild, even if your medications work well, even if you have wonderful doctors — there's a quiet, heavy truth that comes with lupus: your body has turned against you, and even on your best days, trusting it fully can feel impossible. That kind of realization doesn't just sit quietly in the background — it shapes your mental and emotional health in ways that deserve attention and compassion.

For many people with lupus, anxiety and depression are frequent, unwelcome visitors. Sometimes they're a reaction to the stress of living with a disease that's unpredictable and poorly understood. The constant sense of walking on thin ice —

wondering if the next flare is around the corner, worrying about how long your good days will last, second-guessing every new ache or rash — can create a constant undercurrent of anxiety that never fully goes away. There's the anxiety of waiting for test results, of wondering if a symptom is "just lupus" or something more serious, and of knowing that even your doctors may not always have clear answers. There's also the deeper existential anxiety that comes with knowing your health is fragile, that the future you once pictured might need to be rewritten, and that some doors — careers, parenthood, travel, or even carefree spontaneity — might be harder to walk through now.

Depression often rides alongside this anxiety, sometimes quietly and sometimes like a storm. Some of it comes from grieving the life you had before lupus, especially if your symptoms force you to scale back your ambitions, change careers, or step away from hobbies and social activities you loved. It's common to feel a sense of loss, not just for your health, but for your sense of self — who you were when your body wasn't constantly reminding you of its limits. There's also a more biological side to depression in lupus. Inflammation itself can affect the brain, altering the way it processes mood and stress. Lupus flares, especially those involving the central nervous system, can directly trigger chemical changes that make depression feel heavier and harder to shake. It's not all in your head —

your brain and immune system are in constant conversation, and when one is inflamed, the other often suffers.

Then there's the grief — a quieter, more private process that doesn't always get the attention it deserves. A chronic diagnosis like lupus forces you to say goodbye to some of the things you once took for granted: the assumption that your body would always bounce back, that your plans would unfold the way you imagined, that health was something you could control if you just ate right and exercised enough. This grief is complicated because it's not a single event — it's a series of small losses that accumulate over time. Cancelled plans, lost opportunities, friendships that fade because you can't keep up. It's grief for the body you used to have, the freedom you used to feel, the future you once assumed was yours. And because lupus is unpredictable, this grief never fully ends — it ebbs and flows, sometimes flaring up right alongside your physical symptoms, sometimes receding into the background, only to resurface when you're reminded of what's been taken.

Because lupus is invisible to most people, it's easy to feel isolated in this emotional landscape. Friends and family may sympathize at first, but over time, when you still don't "look sick," they may struggle to understand why you're still tired, still cancelling plans, still needing accommodations. Even people who care deeply about you may not fully grasp the constant mental effort it takes to manage symptoms, track medications, advocate for yourself at appointments, and make peace with all the uncertainty. This isolation — the sense that you're living in a reality no one else can fully see — can deepen both anxiety and depression, making it even harder to ask for help.

That's why professional support can be such a lifeline. Therapy isn't just for people in crisis — it's for anyone who needs a safe space to process their emotions, grieve their losses, and develop coping strategies that fit their real lives. A therapist who understands chronic illness can help you navigate the emotional rollercoaster of lupus — the fear, the frustration, the guilt, the grief — and help you learn to separate who you are from what your disease says about you. They can help you untangle the mental knots that form when you start blaming yourself for flares or feeling like you're not "strong enough" to handle lupus perfectly. They can help you set boundaries, communicate your needs to family and friends, and find ways to rebuild your sense of self, even when your body feels unreliable. Sometimes, therapy also helps you recognize when medication for depression or anxiety might be part of the solution — because treating your mind is just as important as treating your immune system.

Beyond professional help, building a strong support network can be just as vital. This doesn't have to mean a huge circle of people — even one or two trusted friends, family members, or fellow patients who really understand can make all the difference. Connecting with others who have lupus, whether through local support groups or online communities, can be especially comforting. There's something uniquely healing about talking to someone who doesn't need you to explain what a flare feels like, who already knows the frustration of invisible symptoms and the exhaustion of endless medical appointments. These connections can help break the isolation, reminding you that you're not the only one navigating this path, and that strength doesn't mean doing it alone.

The emotional side of lupus is just as real — and just as deserving of attention — as the physical symptoms. It's not a sign of weakness to feel anxious, overwhelmed, angry, or sad. It's a sign that you're human, living through something challenging, and doing your best with a body that doesn't always cooperate. Taking care of your mental health isn't a luxury or an afterthought — it's part of your treatment plan, just as important as medications and blood tests. Your mind and body are in this together, and by caring for both, you give yourself the best chance at not just surviving lupus, but living well with it, with all the grace, strength, and resilience you never knew you had — until lupus taught you how much you could endure.

CHAPTER 13: SUN PROTECTION

When you're living with lupus, the sun isn't just a source of warmth and light — it's a potential trigger, one that can quietly stir up trouble both on the surface of your skin and deep inside your body. Sun sensitivity, also called photosensitivity, is incredibly common in people with lupus, and for many, it's one of the first signs that something isn't quite right. A few minutes of sunlight that might leave someone else with a light tan or nothing at all can leave a person with lupus with redness, itching, or rashes that appear hours or even days later. But the effects aren't always limited to the skin — in some people, sun exposure can actually trigger a full-body flare, worsening joint pain, fatigue, and even internal organ inflammation. It's one of the most frustrating parts of living with lupus, especially if you've always loved spending time outdoors, and it can make something as simple as a walk in the park or a family picnic feel risky instead of relaxing.

The reason sunlight is such a problem in lupus has to do with ultraviolet (UV) light — the invisible rays that come from the sun and penetrate deep into your skin. In everyone, UV light causes some degree of cell damage, but in people with lupus, the immune system is already overreactive and primed to misinterpret those damaged skin cells as threats.

When UV rays hit the skin, they damage DNA inside skin cells, and as those damaged cells die off, they release bits of that DNA into the bloodstream. In people with healthy immune systems, the body cleans up that debris quietly. But in people with lupus, the immune system sees that DNA as foreign, treating it like an invader and launching an immune response to attack it. This not only causes skin rashes, but in some cases, it can set off inflammation throughout the body, essentially turning sun exposure into a trigger for a full-on lupus flare.

That's why sun protection isn't just about preventing sunburn — it's a key part of managing your lupus and protecting your overall health. Sunscreen becomes more than just something you slap on at the beach — it becomes an everyday tool to help keep your immune system from overreacting. Not all sunscreens are created equal, though, and people with lupus often need to be extra careful about the kinds they use. Look for sunscreens labeled broad-spectrum, which means they protect against both UVA and UVB rays — both types of UV light can trigger lupus symptoms. A sun protection factor (SPF) of at least 50 is usually recommended, especially if you have skin lupus or have noticed that even brief sun exposure triggers symptoms.

Physical or mineral sunscreens, which contain zinc oxide or titanium dioxide, are often preferred for people with lupus because they sit on top of the skin and physically block UV rays, rather than being absorbed into the skin like chemical sunscreens. They're also less likely to irritate sensitive skin, which is common in lupus. The downside is that mineral sunscreens can sometimes leave a white cast, especially on darker skin tones, but many newer formulations are tinted or designed to blend more easily. Whichever type you choose, generous application is key — most people apply far less sunscreen than they actually need. A good rule of thumb is about a teaspoon for your face and a shot glass full for your whole body, applied at least 15 minutes before going outside. And reapplication matters too — even the best sunscreen wears off after a couple of hours, especially if you're sweating or swimming.

But sunscreen alone isn't enough when you have lupus. Protective clothing adds another layer of defense, and there are now plenty of lightweight, breathable options that are designed specifically for sun protection. Long-sleeved shirts, wide-brimmed hats, and sunglasses with UV protection are all smart investments, especially if you spend a lot of time outdoors. Some clothing is labeled with an Ultraviolet Protection Factor (UPF), which tells you how well the fabric blocks UV rays — look for UPF 50 for the best protection. The nice thing about sun-protective clothing is that you don't have to remember to reapply it, and it protects you even if you're caught outside unexpectedly. Many brands now offer stylish, comfortable options, so you don't have to choose between protection and comfort.

Outdoor safety with lupus is all about planning ahead and stacking layers of protection — sunscreen, clothing, and smart timing. The sun's rays are strongest between 10 a.m. and 4 p.m., so if you can, try to schedule outdoor activities for early morning or late afternoon, when the sun is lower and less intense. Shade is your friend, whether it's a tree, an umbrella, or a wide-brimmed hat — any barrier between you and direct sunlight helps. If you're going to be outside for a while, bring extra sunscreen, so you can reapply without having to hunt for a store. And always listen to your body — if you start to feel fatigued, dizzy, or notice your skin getting red or irritated, head indoors right away. Even small amounts of UV exposure can trigger symptoms in some people with lupus, so erring on the side of caution is always smart.

It's natural to feel frustrated about these limits, especially if you used to love spending time in the sun. It can feel unfair to have to think so much about something other people take for granted — a day at the beach, a hike, or even just sitting outside at a café. But protecting yourself from the sun doesn't mean you have to give up on enjoying life outdoors. With some adjustments, some creativity, and the right tools, you can still spend time outside — just in a way that keeps your lupus quiet and your body safe. Think of sun protection not as a restriction, but as an act of self-care, a way of respecting your body's needs and protecting yourself for the long haul. The sun may be beautiful, but for people with lupus, shade, sunscreen, and smart choices are even more beautiful — because they help keep you healthy, strong, and in control, no matter what the sun tries to do.

CHAPTER 14: PREGNANCY AND LUPUS

For anyone thinking about pregnancy, it's a time filled with excitement, questions, and maybe a little anxiety. But when you have lupus, that mix of emotions can feel even more intense. You might wonder whether it's even safe to get pregnant, or if lupus will automatically make pregnancy high-risk. You might worry about how your medications will affect the baby, or whether pregnancy could make your lupus worse. These are all valid concerns — but the good news is that most people with lupus can have safe, healthy pregnancies, especially with careful planning, the right medical team, and a solid understanding of how lupus and pregnancy interact. Lupus may complicate the path to parenthood, but it doesn't close the door entirely — and understanding what to expect can make that path feel much more manageable.

The first and most important piece of advice for anyone with lupus who's thinking about pregnancy is this: timing matters. The best time to try for a baby is when your lupus has been quiet for at least six months, meaning no active flares and stable organ function, particularly in the kidneys. Pregnancy itself is a stress test on the body, and if your lupus is already flaring when you get pregnant, the risk of complications — both for you and the baby — rises significantly. A healthy pregnancy starts long before conception, with a thorough checkup from your rheumatologist and obstetrician, ideally one who specializes in high-risk or maternal-fetal medicine. Together, they can help you assess your current lupus activity, review your medications, and develop a plan to ensure your body is in the best possible shape before you even see those two pink lines.

One of the biggest concerns for people with lupus who are pregnant — or hoping to become pregnant — is medication safety. Many lupus medications are safe to continue during pregnancy, but some need to be adjusted or stopped because they could harm the developing baby. Hydroxychloroquine is generally considered safe and even beneficial during pregnancy, as it helps reduce flare risk and may even lower the chance of complications like lupus nephritis or pre-eclampsia. Other medications, like azathioprine, can also be continued safely in many cases. But some commonly used lupus drugs — including mycophenolate mofetil (CellCept), methotrexate, and cyclophosphamide — are known to cause birth defects or pregnancy loss, and need to be stopped well before conception. This is why planning ahead is so important — your doctor can help you transition to safer medications and monitor how your body responds to those changes before you get pregnant. The goal is always to find a balance between controlling your lupus and keeping the baby safe, and with the right adjustments, that balance is very possible.

Once you're pregnant, your doctors will monitor you more closely than someone without lupus, because pregnancy does bring some additional risks. One of the biggest concerns is pre-eclampsia, a dangerous condition marked by high blood pressure, protein in the urine, and organ stress, which is more common in people with lupus nephritis or a history of kidney problems. Regular blood pressure checks, urine tests, and blood work help catch any signs of trouble early, giving your doctors a chance to intervene before it becomes serious. There's also a slightly higher risk of preterm birth, low birth weight, and fetal growth restriction, so frequent ultrasounds may be part of your care plan to track the baby's growth and development.

Another concern for some people with lupus is antiphospholipid syndrome (APS), a condition where the immune system produces antibodies that increase the risk of blood clots and pregnancy complications like miscarriage or stillbirth. If you have antiphospholipid antibodies, your doctor may recommend taking low-dose aspirin or even heparin injections throughout your pregnancy to reduce clotting risk and improve blood flow to the placenta. These medications, while intimidating at first, are proven to improve pregnancy outcomes, and they're a common part of lupus pregnancy care.

For a small number of people with lupus, particularly those who test positive for anti-Ro or anti-La antibodies, there's also a small risk of a condition called neonatal lupus, which can affect the baby's skin, liver, or blood cells temporarily after birth. In rare cases, these antibodies can also cause a condition called congenital heart block, where the baby's heart develops an abnormal rhythm. It sounds frightening, but the good news is that most babies born to mothers with lupus are completely healthy, and doctors have protocols in place to monitor for these rare complications during pregnancy, including regular fetal heart monitoring starting around 16 weeks. If any concerns arise, your medical team can work with pediatric specialists to plan for the baby's care after birth. Most cases of neonatal lupus — especially the skin and blood-related ones — resolve on their own within a few months, and lifelong complications are extremely rare.

The postpartum period — those first few months after delivery — is a critical time for anyone with lupus. The shift in hormones, combined with the physical demands of caring for a newborn, can increase the risk of a lupus flare. This isn't inevitable, but it's common enough that doctors generally recommend close follow-up after delivery, including regular blood work and check-ins with your rheumatologist. Fatigue is part of life with a new baby, but if your exhaustion feels crushing, or if joint pain, skin rashes, or other lupus symptoms start creeping back, don't brush it off as just the normal challenges of motherhood. Postpartum flares are real, but they're also manageable, especially if they're caught early. Having a plan in place before delivery, including adjustments to medications if needed, can help make the transition smoother and reduce the risk of serious complications.

Through all of this — the planning, the appointments, the careful balancing of risks and benefits — it's important to remember that people with lupus have healthy babies every day. Lupus may make pregnancy more complicated, but it doesn't make it impossible. The key is being proactive, building a strong team of supportive doctors, and listening to your body every step of the way. Whether you're dreaming of your first baby or hoping to expand your family, lupus doesn't have to take that dream away. With good planning, careful monitoring, and the right care team by your side, you can navigate pregnancy and parenthood with lupus — not perfectly, not without challenges, but with strength, knowledge, and confidence in yourself and your body.

CHAPTER 15: LIVING WITH LUPUS AT WORK AND SCHOOL

Living with lupus means carrying your health with you everywhere — not just to doctor's appointments, but into every corner of your life, including work and school. Whether you're sitting in a classroom, working in an office, or pursuing a career in something physically demanding, lupus is always there in the background, affecting your energy levels, your focus, your ability to plan ahead, and sometimes your confidence. Lupus isn't always visible to the people around you, which can make navigating work or school even more complicated, because the struggles you face every day might be completely invisible to your coworkers, classmates, teachers, or supervisors. Whether you're dealing with crushing fatigue in the middle of a workday, trying to study for an exam while nursing sore joints, or wondering how much to tell your boss or professor about your diagnosis, balancing lupus with work or school is a challenge that takes patience, creativity, and a willingness to advocate for yourself — even when you'd rather blend into the background.

One of the biggest hurdles at both work and school is managing fatigue and flares while still meeting deadlines and keeping up with responsibilities.

Lupus fatigue is a different beast from ordinary tiredness — it's unpredictable, often overwhelming, and doesn't always improve with rest. On days when you're exhausted before the day even starts, the idea of sitting through a long meeting, finishing a project, or making it to every class can feel impossible. The same goes for lupus flares, which don't follow schedules or deadlines. A project might be due the same week your joints swell up so badly you can't type. An exam might land right in the middle of a flare that leaves you too foggy to concentrate. The unpredictable nature of lupus means that even when you plan well, your body doesn't always cooperate, and learning how to adapt without guilt is one of the most important survival skills you can develop.

At work, this often means pacing yourself whenever possible. If your job allows some flexibility, consider spreading demanding tasks across the day rather than stacking them all at once. Breaks — even short ones to stretch, breathe, or rest your eyes — can make a big difference in preserving your energy. If you work on a computer, ergonomic adjustments like a supportive chair, wrist supports, and screen adjustments can reduce the physical strain on your body, especially if you deal with joint pain or stiffness. Learning to recognize your own early warning signs — like increased fatigue, subtle joint stiffness, or cognitive fog — can help you take steps to dial back your workload before a full-blown flare makes it impossible to keep up.

Navigating disability protections and accommodations at work can feel intimidating, especially if you're worried about being judged or treated differently. But in many countries, including the United States, lupus is legally recognized as a disability under laws like the Americans with Disabilities Act (ADA), which means you're entitled to reasonable accommodations that allow you to do your job without compromising your health. These accommodations might include things like flexible work hours, the ability to work from home during flares, adjustments to your physical workspace, or even permission to take extra breaks when needed. Requesting accommodations doesn't mean you're asking for special treatment — it means you're asking for the support you need to keep doing your job effectively, without sacrificing your health. If you're unsure how to start the conversation, a letter from your doctor explaining how lupus affects you can help open the door, and many companies have human resources departments that are experienced in working with employees who have chronic illnesses.

For students, the challenges can be even trickier because school schedules tend to be rigid, with fixed class times, exams on set dates, and a culture that often rewards pushing through at all costs. But just like in the workplace, students with lupus are often eligible for accommodations through their school's disability services office. These accommodations can include extra time on exams, permission to record lectures if taking notes by hand is difficult, flexible attendance policies for flares, or even remote learning options during periods when getting to campus isn't possible. The key is to advocate for yourself early, ideally as soon as you're diagnosed or when symptoms start interfering with your ability to keep up with your classes. Many schools have confidential disability services departments that work directly with students to create personalized accommodation plans, and you don't need to tell your professors every detail about your health if you're not comfortable — the school handles the communication, ensuring your privacy is protected.

Balancing schoolwork with health management also requires a lot of flexibility and self-compassion. You might need to break studying into shorter sessions, prioritize sleep over cramming, or ask classmates for notes when you have to miss class. Group projects, presentations, and long exams can all be physically and mentally draining, so building in recovery time around those high-demand periods can help protect you from crashing afterward. If you're in college or university, consider building a schedule that gives you gaps between classes to rest, eat, or just breathe, rather than stacking back-to-back commitments that leave you no room to recover.

Whether you're at work or school, one of the hardest things about lupus is figuring out how much to share about your diagnosis. There's no universal rule — some people feel comfortable being open about their condition, while others prefer to keep it private. What matters most is that you feel in control of the narrative, sharing only what's necessary to get the support you need. In some workplaces or schools, education can be powerful — explaining that lupus is an autoimmune disease, not contagious, and that symptoms can be invisible might help foster understanding and empathy. In other situations, you might decide that it's enough to say you have a chronic health condition without getting into the details. There's no right or wrong — it's about finding what level of disclosure feels safe and empowering for you.

Most importantly, remember that having lupus doesn't mean you don't belong at work or school. You deserve the same opportunities to pursue your education, your career, and your dreams as anyone else — you just need to approach it in a way that works with your body, not against it. That means honoring your limits, asking for help when you need it, and understanding that needing accommodations or flexibility isn't a failure — it's a necessary part of thriving with a chronic illness. You are not less capable, less worthy, or less valuable because of your lupus. If anything, the resilience, adaptability, and problem-solving skills you develop as you learn to balance your health with your ambitions will make you even more prepared for the challenges life throws your way. With the right support, smart strategies, and a willingness to listen to your body, you can build a career, earn your degree, and achieve your goals — not despite lupus, but alongside it, as someone who knows how to persevere with grace and grit.

CHAPTER 16: LUPUS IN CHILDREN AND TEENS

Lupus is difficult enough for adults, but when it strikes children or teenagers, it adds an entirely different layer of complexity — for the young patients themselves, for their parents, and for their teachers, classmates, and friends. While lupus can occur at any age, when it shows up in childhood or adolescence, it tends to behave a little differently than the version seen in adults. Pediatric lupus, as it's often called, is usually more aggressive, more likely to involve the kidneys, brain, and other organs, and can be harder to get into remission. Children's immune systems are still developing when lupus strikes, which may be part of the reason their disease tends to be more severe. But children also have something adults with lupus don't — the ability to grow up with a sense of resilience, adaptability, and self-advocacy skills that can shape the way they manage their health for the rest of their lives.

For children and teens, the diagnosis itself can be bewildering. Most kids have never heard of lupus before, and explaining a disease where your own immune system turns against you isn't easy, especially when symptoms vary from day to day. One day, a child with lupus might feel well enough to play soccer or go to a birthday party, and the next day, they might be too exhausted to get out of bed. That unpredictability is hard for anyone to live with, but for children and teens, who crave consistency, independence, and fitting in, it can feel especially unfair. Young patients often struggle to understand why their bodies feel like a battleground and why their treatment involves so many doctors' appointments, blood draws, medications, and rules about sun protection, rest, and avoiding infections. For teenagers, who are naturally pulling away from parents and developing their own identity, needing constant medical care and family involvement in health decisions can feel particularly suffocating — even if it's necessary.

Helping children and teens cope emotionally with lupus starts with giving them age-appropriate information. Younger children don't need to know every medical detail, but they do need to understand that lupus isn't contagious, that it's not their fault, and that their doctors and parents are working as a team to help them feel better. Explaining lupus in simple terms — that their immune system is a little confused and needs extra help to work properly — can make it less scary. For teenagers, honesty is key, and giving them a role in their care, whether it's keeping track of their medications, writing down symptoms in a journal, or asking questions at doctor visits, can help them feel more in control. Adolescence is a time when most teens are starting to define who they are — what they like, what they want to do, how they want to be seen — and lupus can feel like an uninvited intrusion into that process. Helping teens separate who they are from their diagnosis — reminding them that lupus is part of their life, but not their whole identity — can be empowering, especially when they feel like they've lost control of their body.

At school, challenges often multiply, because lupus doesn't always follow the school calendar. Fatigue, joint pain, brain fog, and flares can make it difficult to keep up with assignments, participate in gym class, or sit through a full day of classes. Some children and teens with lupus need individualized education plans (IEPs) or 504 plans, which are legal agreements that outline specific accommodations to help them succeed academically. These accommodations might include extra time for assignments and exams, permission to leave class to rest, flexible attendance policies, or access to online learning during periods when lupus symptoms make it impossible to be in school. Working with school administrators and teachers to create a supportive environment can make an enormous difference — but only if parents and students feel comfortable advocating for what they need.

One of the hardest parts for young people with lupus is feeling different from their peers. Children and teens often want to blend in, and having a chronic illness that requires constant attention — from medications to sun precautions to unpredictable absences — can make them feel like they stand out in all the wrong ways. This can lead to feelings of isolation, frustration, and even resentment, especially if their friends don't understand why they're always tired or why they have to skip certain activities. Encouraging open conversations with friends, either directly or with the help of a supportive adult, can help break down some of those walls. Sometimes it's as simple as explaining that lupus is an autoimmune condition that makes the immune system overreact and that it's not contagious or anyone's fault. When friends understand even a little bit, they're often more supportive and less likely to make insensitive comments — and sometimes they become fierce advocates for their friend with lupus.

Connecting young lupus patients with peer support — other children or teens who also have lupus — can be transformative. Knowing they're not the only one going through this experience can help them feel less alone and more understood. Many hospitals and lupus organizations offer support groups, online forums, and special camps for young people with autoimmune diseases, creating safe spaces where they can ask questions, share their frustrations, and just be themselves without having to explain every little thing about their health. Seeing other young people thrive despite lupus can also be incredibly encouraging, showing them that life with lupus can still include friendships, sports, hobbies, travel, college, and all the other milestones they dream about.

For parents, the balancing act can feel impossible at times — trying to protect your child's health while also letting them have as normal a childhood as possible. It's natural to want to shield them from anything that might trigger a flare, but it's also important to let them live their lives — to play, to laugh, to test limits, and to feel like kids or teenagers, not just patients. This balance will look different for every family, and it often changes over time as children learn to manage their symptoms and become more confident in advocating for themselves. The goal isn't to pretend lupus doesn't exist, but to make room for joy and possibility, even in the middle of medical uncertainty.

Lupus in children and teens is undeniably challenging, but with the right support, good communication, and a team approach, young people with lupus can grow up to be resilient, empowered adults who understand their bodies, advocate for their needs, and embrace their lives fully — not in spite of lupus, but with the strength and wisdom that comes from learning to live with it from such a young age. Childhood and adolescence might be different with lupus, but they can still be filled with growth, discovery, connection, and hope — and those are the things that truly matter.

CHAPTER 17: COMPLEMENTARY AND ALTERNATIVE THERAPIES: WHAT HELPS, WHAT'S HYPE

When you're living with lupus, it's natural to wonder if there's something — anything — outside of your regular medications that might help. The internet is filled with stories, suggestions, and bold claims about alternative therapies, some promising to ease symptoms, others going so far as to claim they can cure lupus altogether. It's tempting to hope that something natural, something gentler than immunosuppressants and steroids, might make a real difference. But sorting through what might actually help and what's nothing more than false hope wrapped in pseudoscience can be tricky, especially when you're tired, frustrated, and just want to feel better. The truth is, complementary and alternative therapies do have a place in lupus care for many people — but they should be tools to support your treatment, not replace it. Knowing which approaches are worth trying and which ones to avoid can help you make informed, confident choices about your health.

One area with growing research support is mind-body approaches, therapies that focus on the connection between your mind, your emotions, and your physical health. Living with lupus is incredibly stressful — the unpredictability, the flares, the never-ending appointments and blood work — and that stress isn't just unpleasant. It actually has the power to make inflammation worse, setting off hormonal changes that push your immune system into overdrive. That's why techniques that help calm the nervous system, like meditation, guided imagery, and deep breathing exercises, can be surprisingly helpful. These practices don't magically erase lupus symptoms, but they help lower stress hormones like cortisol, which may help reduce flare frequency and severity over time. They also provide a sense of control, something that's easy to lose when you're living with a disease as unpredictable as lupus. Even just a few minutes a day of focused breathing, quiet meditation, or gentle visualization can create a buffer between you and the stress that often accompanies chronic illness.

Acupuncture is another mind-body therapy that some people with lupus turn to, especially for managing pain, fatigue, and stress. Acupuncture involves inserting very thin needles into specific points on the body, based on principles from traditional Chinese medicine. While the scientific evidence on acupuncture for lupus is limited, some research suggests it may help with pain management and stress reduction, especially for joint pain and muscle tension. If you're considering acupuncture, it's important to choose a licensed, experienced practitioner, ideally one who has experience working with people who have autoimmune diseases. It's also important to make sure your acupuncturist understands your medications, especially if you're on blood thinners, which can increase the risk of bleeding.

Supplements and herbal remedies are another area where curiosity often leads people to experiment, sometimes with good results, sometimes with frustration, and occasionally with real danger. It's easy to assume that anything labeled "natural" must be safe, but natural doesn't always mean harmless — especially when you have an autoimmune disease and are already taking powerful medications. Some supplements have some evidence behind them for supporting health in lupus, while others have either no proof at all or could actually interfere with your medications or worsen your disease.

For example, omega-3 fatty acids, found in fish oil, have shown some benefit in reducing inflammation in autoimmune diseases, including lupus. They're not a substitute for medications, but they may offer modest improvements in joint pain and inflammation, especially if your diet is low in omega-3s. Vitamin D is another supplement worth discussing with your doctor, especially since many people with lupus avoid the sun, which is the body's main way of producing vitamin D. Low vitamin D levels have been linked to worse disease activity, so correcting a deficiency could help support your immune system and bone health. Calcium is also important if you're on steroids, which can weaken bones over time.

On the other hand, some herbal remedies that are widely promoted for general health can be risky for people with lupus. Echinacea, for example, is often marketed as an immune booster, but the very last thing you want with lupus is to stimulate an already overactive immune system. Similarly, alfalfa sprouts — often recommended as a "superfood" — can actually trigger lupus flares because they contain a compound that may activate the immune system. High-dose turmeric, sometimes promoted as an anti-inflammatory herb, may interfere with blood clotting, which could be dangerous if you already have antiphospholipid syndrome or are on blood thinners. Even supplements that seem harmless, like herbal teas or detox blends, can sometimes contain ingredients that interact with your medications or overstimulate your immune system.

The biggest red flag in the world of alternative therapies is anyone promising a cure for lupus. There is no cure for lupus — not in mainstream medicine, and not in alternative medicine either. Anyone claiming they can cure lupus with a special diet, a secret supplement, a detox cleanse, or an exotic herbal blend is not being honest with you. These claims prey on people's fear, frustration, and hope, and they often come with a high price tag — both financially and in terms of your health if they cause you to delay or abandon treatments that actually work. The best way to spot false cures is to be wary of anything that sounds too good to be true, especially if it comes with testimonials instead of scientific evidence, and if it encourages you to stop your prescribed medications.

That doesn't mean you have to give up on exploring complementary therapies — it just means doing so with your eyes open, working in partnership with your doctors, and treating these therapies as add-ons, not replacements, for proven treatments. The best approach is to keep your medical team in the loop about anything you're trying — even if it's just a supplement or a new type of massage — because some therapies that seem harmless can affect how your medications work or increase your risk of side effects.

Ultimately, the goal of complementary therapies isn't to replace your medications or erase your diagnosis — it's to help you feel better, cope better, and live better, with fewer side effects and more tools to manage pain, stress, and fatigue. Some therapies, like meditation or gentle yoga, can become part of your daily routine, while others might be occasional tools you reach for when your symptoms are particularly tough. The key is balance — using both conventional medicine and complementary approaches together, in a way that supports your whole self — body, mind, and spirit — without falling for quick fixes or false hope.

With the right mix of trustworthy information, open communication with your medical team, and careful experimentation, you can build a toolbox of complementary strategies that truly support your lupus journey — not with empty promises, but with practical tools that help you feel stronger, calmer, and more in control, one step at a time.

CHAPTER 18: VACCINES, INFECTIONS, AND LUPUS

When you live with lupus, infections aren't just inconvenient — they can be dangerous. Even a simple cold, a stomach bug, or a mild urinary tract infection can throw your immune system into confusion, leading not only to typical infection symptoms like fever and fatigue but also to a full-blown lupus flare. This happens because your immune system is already overreactive, primed to respond too aggressively to anything it sees as a threat — including viruses, bacteria, and other infections. That overreaction can spill over into attacking your own tissues, causing your joints to swell, your skin to break out in rashes, or your kidneys or lungs to become inflamed. It's one of the most frustrating parts of living with lupus — sometimes it's not the infection itself that causes the most trouble, but your body's over-the-top response to it. This is why infection prevention becomes an essential part of managing lupus, not just for your comfort but to protect your long-term health.

One of the simplest, most effective ways to protect yourself from infections is through vaccination — but when you have lupus, the question of which vaccines are safe becomes a little more complicated.

Vaccines work by training your immune system to recognize and fight off future infections, but for people with lupus — especially those on immunosuppressants — not all vaccines are equally safe or effective. In general, inactivated vaccines, which contain killed viruses or bacteria, are considered safe for people with lupus. This includes flu shots, pneumococcal vaccines (to prevent pneumonia), COVID-19 vaccines, and hepatitis vaccines. These vaccines don't contain live germs, so they can't cause infection — even in someone with a weakened immune system — and they help protect against illnesses that could trigger flares or cause severe complications.

On the other hand, live vaccines, which contain weakened but still living viruses, are more complicated. These include vaccines for measles, mumps, rubella (MMR), chickenpox (varicella), shingles, and some types of yellow fever vaccines. In people with healthy immune systems, these live vaccines don't cause illness, but in people whose immune systems are suppressed — either by lupus itself or by medications like steroids, methotrexate, mycophenolate, or biologics — live vaccines can pose a small risk of triggering infection. That doesn't mean they're always forbidden — sometimes the risks of skipping a vaccine outweigh the risks of getting it — but it does mean the decision needs to be made carefully in consultation with your rheumatologist or infectious disease specialist. In some cases, you might be able to get a live vaccine if your lupus is well-controlled and you're not on heavy immunosuppressants, but in other cases, it might be safer to rely on indirect protection, like ensuring your family members and close contacts are vaccinated so they're less likely to pass infections to you.

Timing also matters when it comes to vaccines and lupus. If your lupus is in flare, your immune system may not respond as well to a vaccine, meaning you might not get the same level of protection you would if your lupus were quiet. Ideally, vaccines should be given when your disease is stable, and not immediately after starting a new immunosuppressive medication if it can be avoided. That's why vaccination planning should always be part of your long-term lupus care, not just something you think about during flu season. If you're preparing for travel, especially to places where certain vaccines are required, it's worth discussing well in advance with your doctors to make sure you have time to get any necessary vaccines safely.

Even with careful prevention, infections still happen, and when they do, knowing how to respond can make all the difference. The first and most important rule is don't wait too long to seek care. Infections in people with lupus can escalate quickly, especially if you're on medications that suppress your immune system. A low-grade fever, a little cough, or mild urinary symptoms might not seem like a big deal, but in someone with lupus, those small signs can be the first warning of something more serious. Call your doctor if you develop fever, chills, worsening fatigue, cough, shortness of breath, painful urination, or any other symptom that could indicate an infection — even if you think it's nothing. Early treatment can often prevent more serious complications, and in some cases, treating an infection quickly can also help prevent a lupus flare triggered by the infection.

If you do get sick, it's also important to adjust your medications if necessary. Some immunosuppressants may need to be paused temporarily while your body fights off an infection, because they could make it harder for your immune system to clear the germs. On the other hand, abruptly stopping steroids can trigger a flare or adrenal crisis, so any changes to your medications should always be made under the guidance of your doctor. Your rheumatologist and primary care doctor may work together to strike the right balance between controlling your lupus and giving your immune system enough flexibility to fight off the infection.

During an illness, self-care matters more than ever. Rest becomes non-negotiable, even if you feel pressure to push through work, school, or family responsibilities. Staying hydrated helps your body process medications and flush out infections, and simple things like cool compresses for fevers or warm tea for a cough can offer comfort while your body recovers. But the most important part of self-care when you're sick is listening to your body and being willing to ask for help — whether that's from your doctors, your family, or your employer. Lupus already asks a lot of your body, and when you add an infection into the mix, giving yourself grace and time to heal isn't weakness — it's essential.

Living with lupus means thinking about infections in a way most people never have to, but with the right combination of vaccines, smart prevention strategies, early intervention, and self-care, you can reduce the risk of serious infections and their complications. It's not about living in fear — it's about being proactive, knowing your risks, and using all the tools available to stay safe, stay well, and stay ahead of both infections and lupus itself. You can't avoid every virus or bacteria, but you can give your body the best chance to handle them when they come — and that's one of the most powerful ways to take control of your health with lupus.

CHAPTER 19: BUILDING YOUR HEALTHCARE TEAM

Managing lupus isn't something you do alone. It's not a condition that can be handled by just one doctor or one type of specialist. Instead, living well with lupus means building a healthcare team — a group of professionals who each bring their own expertise, working together to give you the best possible care. Lupus affects so many different parts of the body, and the symptoms can change from year to year, or even month to month. That's why having the right team in place — a team you trust, who know you well, and who communicate with each other — can make all the difference between feeling overwhelmed and feeling confident that your health is in good hands.

At the center of your team is your rheumatologist, the specialist who understands autoimmune diseases like lupus inside and out. Your rheumatologist is the quarterback of your care — the person who helps you navigate the big picture, deciding when to start or stop medications, monitoring your overall disease activity, and coordinating care with your other specialists when needed. Your rheumatologist is usually the one who orders your regular blood work, keeps track of any new symptoms, and works with you to adjust your treatment plan over time. Because lupus can be so unpredictable, having a strong, trusting relationship with your rheumatologist is essential. They're not just there to prescribe medication — they're there to listen to your concerns, help you understand your options, and work with you to make decisions that fit your life, not just your lab results.

But your rheumatologist can't do it all alone, and depending on how lupus affects you, there may be times when you need to bring in other specialists to address specific organs or symptoms. If lupus affects your kidneys, you'll need a nephrologist, a kidney specialist who can help monitor your kidney function, interpret urine tests and biopsies, and recommend kidney-specific treatments if you develop lupus nephritis. Nephrologists play an especially important role in preserving kidney function over the long term, making sure any damage is caught early and treated aggressively to prevent permanent kidney disease.

If your lupus involves your skin — whether it's the classic butterfly rash, discoid lesions, or sun sensitivity — you may also need a dermatologist who's experienced in treating autoimmune skin conditions. A dermatologist can help with special creams, light treatments, and medications targeted specifically at skin symptoms, and they can work with your rheumatologist to make sure your skin symptoms aren't signs of a broader flare.

If lupus touches your heart, lungs, or blood vessels, a cardiologist may become part of your team. People with lupus have a higher risk of developing heart disease, pericarditis, pleuritis, and blood clots, so having a cardiologist who understands autoimmune disease can be incredibly valuable. They can monitor your blood pressure, cholesterol, and heart function, and they can work with your other doctors to make sure your medications are protecting both your lupus and your heart. In some cases, a pulmonologist, a lung specialist, may also be involved if you develop lung inflammation or scarring.

Even though your lupus care revolves around specialists, your primary care doctor still plays a crucial role. They're often the first line of defense for things like routine screenings, infections, vaccinations, and general health concerns that aren't directly related to lupus. They help coordinate care between your specialists, and they're often the person you turn to for day-to-day health questions — from coughs and colds to managing high blood pressure or cholesterol. They're also in a good position to see the big picture, making sure your overall health — not just your lupus — is being cared for. A strong relationship with your primary care provider helps ensure that nothing falls through the cracks, especially when you have a lot of moving parts in your care.

Your pharmacist is also an often-overlooked but incredibly valuable member of your team. With lupus, you may be on multiple medications, each with its own potential side effects and interactions. Your pharmacist can help you understand your medications, including when and how to take them, what side effects to watch for, and how they might interact with over-the-counter drugs, supplements, or herbal remedies. If you ever feel unsure about your medications — whether they're working, whether they're safe to take together, or whether a new symptom might be related to a drug — your pharmacist is a great person to turn to for clear, practical advice.

Because nutrition can play a role in managing lupus symptoms — especially inflammation, bone health, and heart health — a nutritionist or dietitian with experience in autoimmune disease can also be a helpful ally. They can work with you to develop a balanced, anti-inflammatory eating plan, making sure you're getting enough calcium, vitamin D, and other nutrients you need, especially if you're on steroids or have kidney involvement. They can also help you navigate dietary changes if you develop food sensitivities, weight changes, or digestive symptoms related to lupus or your medications.

Finally, mental health professionals — whether it's a therapist, counselor, psychologist, or psychiatrist — are just as important as your physical health team.

Living with lupus can take a serious emotional toll, from the stress of unpredictable symptoms to the grief of losing the life you imagined for yourself. A mental health professional can help you cope with anxiety, depression, health-related stress, and the emotional weight of living with a chronic illness. They can also teach coping skills, help you navigate difficult conversations with family or employers, and help you build resilience so that lupus doesn't dominate your sense of who you are. There's no shame in needing emotional support — in fact, recognizing when you need help is a sign of strength and self-awareness.

Your healthcare team might start small — just you, your rheumatologist, and maybe your primary care doctor — but over time, as your lupus journey evolves, your team may grow and shift to match your needs. What matters most is that your team works together, with open communication and shared goals, centered around your quality of life. It's not about collecting specialists just for the sake of it — it's about building a network of professionals who understand you, your body, your values, and your hopes, and who work together to help you live as fully and comfortably as possible, with lupus along for the ride but never in the driver's seat.

The best care happens when you are at the center, actively involved in the conversations, asking questions, voicing your concerns, and making sure that every member of your team sees you as a whole person, not just a diagnosis. With the right people by your side, you're not just managing lupus — you're building a life that works for you, supported by experts who respect your voice and your experience every step of the way.

CHAPTER 20: CHECKLIST FOR EVERYDAY LUPUS CARE

Living with lupus means learning to live in partnership with your body, even when it feels unpredictable and unreliable. Every day brings a new negotiation between what you want to do and what your body will allow. Some days you'll feel almost normal — other days, even getting out of bed can feel like too much. Because lupus doesn't follow a clear schedule, and because symptoms can creep up quietly before exploding into full flares, everyday care isn't just about taking your medications and going to your appointments — it's about staying tuned in to your body, catching small changes early, and being prepared to shift gears when necessary. It's not always easy, but having a simple daily checklist — a personalized framework you can follow without overthinking — can help you feel more in control, even on the most chaotic days.

At the heart of your everyday lupus care is daily symptom tracking — a habit that might feel tedious at first but can become one of your most powerful tools for understanding your own version of lupus. Tracking your symptoms doesn't have to mean writing an essay every day — even something as simple as rating your fatigue, joint pain, rashes, and mood on a scale of 1 to 10 can help you spot patterns over time. Maybe you notice your joint pain flares up after stressful days, or your fatigue gets worse a few days after sun exposure. Maybe certain foods seem to trigger stomach upset, or you start to see a link between weather changes and flares. These patterns are invisible unless you track them, but once you do, they can help you and your doctors fine-tune your treatment plan, and they can help you recognize early warning signs that a flare might be coming. There are plenty of apps that make tracking easy, but even a simple notebook works if you prefer paper. What matters isn't the format — it's the habit of checking in with yourself regularly, not just during bad flares, but on the quiet days too.

Right alongside symptom tracking is your medication routine, another cornerstone of daily lupus care. Lupus treatment often involves several different medications, each with its own schedule, and missing doses — even occasionally — can make flares more likely. Some medications, like hydroxychloroquine, work best when taken consistently over months or years. Others, like steroids, need to be weaned gradually, and skipping doses can lead to serious problems. That's why building a reliable system for medication reminders is so important. Whether it's a simple pill organizer, a phone alarm, or a dedicated app that tracks doses and refills, the goal is to make sure your medications are part of your daily rhythm, not something you have to actively remember every time. If side effects make it hard to stick with a medication — nausea, dizziness, headaches — tracking those side effects is just as important as tracking symptoms. The sooner you flag them to your doctor, the sooner adjustments can be made.

Another key piece of everyday lupus care is being prepared for doctor visits, so you get the most out of your limited time with your medical team. It's easy to forget questions when you're sitting in the exam room — especially if you're feeling anxious or brain fog is clouding your thinking — so having a running list of questions in your phone or notebook helps ensure nothing important gets missed. These questions can be simple:

- "Is my current medication dose still right for me?"
- "What labs are we checking today and why?"
- "Are there any new treatment options I should know about?"
- "How can I manage this fatigue better?"
- "Should I be concerned about this new symptom?"

The more prepared you are, the more you can partner with your doctor instead of just passively receiving information. You're the expert in your own body — your doctor is the expert in treating lupus — and your best care happens when you work together. Bringing your symptom log to appointments can also help your doctor see patterns you might not notice, and it can help guide decisions about adjusting medications, ordering tests, or referring you to other specialists.

Finally, every person with lupus needs a personalized flare plan, a simple step-by-step guide for what to do when symptoms spike. Flares are part of life with lupus — they're not a sign you've failed or done something wrong, just a sign that your disease is acting up. The goal of a flare plan is to catch flares early, manage symptoms effectively at home when possible, and know when to escalate to your doctor or emergency care. Your flare plan might include:

- Recognizing early signs — increased fatigue, a low-grade fever, new rashes, or swollen joints.
- First steps — rest, hydration, heat or ice packs, adjusting activity levels.
- Medication adjustments — do you need a temporary steroid boost? Are you allowed to increase pain medication?
- When to call your doctor — if new symptoms appear, if symptoms last longer than a set period (like 48 hours), or if you have signs of infection (fever, cough, urinary symptoms).
- Emergency signs — chest pain, shortness of breath, severe headache, sudden vision changes, or any symptom that feels dramatically worse than usual.

It can be helpful to write your flare plan down and keep a copy in your phone, share it with your family or close friends, and review it periodically with your doctor to make sure it's still up to date. Flares are scary, but they're also manageable when you have a clear plan in place, and knowing what to do ahead of time can reduce panic and confusion when symptoms escalate.

Daily lupus care isn't about perfection — it's about creating gentle, flexible routines that help you stay ahead of symptoms, rather than always reacting to them. Some days you'll check every box — you'll track symptoms, take your meds on time, and feel on top of your care. Other days, simply getting through the day is enough, and that's okay too. The goal is to create a foundation of self-awareness and self-care that supports you even on the hardest days, and that empowers you to work with your body instead of fighting against it. With time, these habits become second nature — not just tasks on a checklist, but small, daily acts of self-respect, reminders that you are not powerless, even in the face of a disease as unpredictable as lupus.

Lupus may change the way you live your life, but with a personalized plan, strong habits, and the right support, it doesn't have to define it. You are more than your symptoms, more than your flares, more than your medications — you are someone learning, adapting, and thriving in ways you never expected. And with a little structure and a lot of self-compassion, you can build a life that works for you, one day, one checklist, one small act of care at a time.

CHAPTER 21: YOUR LUPUS ROADMAP: BUILDING A PERSONALIZED ACTION PLAN

Lupus is not a one-size-fits-all disease, and living with it means learning that your version of lupus is as individual as your fingerprint. No two people's symptoms, triggers, or flares look exactly the same, which is why the most powerful tool you can develop is a personalized action plan — a roadmap that helps you navigate your own unique experience with the disease. Doctors provide medications and treatments, but you're the one living in your body every day. You're the one who notices how your symptoms shift with the weather, how stress makes your joints ache, how a certain stretch of good sleep or a dietary change makes you feel just a little better. Putting all of that together into a plan — one that fits your body, your life, your responsibilities, and your goals — helps transform lupus care from something that happens to you into something you're actively shaping. It's not about controlling every symptom or preventing every flare, but about understanding your patterns and working with your body, instead of always feeling at its mercy.

The first step in building your personal lupus roadmap is understanding your own lupus pattern, which takes time, attention, and sometimes a little detective work. Lupus can affect so many different organs, and symptoms often shift over time — what flares up in your twenties may settle down in your thirties, only to be replaced by new challenges. Tracking your flares, symptoms, medications, and lifestyle choices helps you piece together your personal triggers and warning signs. Maybe you notice your fatigue always spikes before a flare, or that stress at work leaves you with joint pain two days later. Maybe certain foods seem to aggravate your symptoms, or maybe you do best when you maintain a certain activity-rest balance. There's no universal lupus pattern, but every person has their own unique rhythm, and the more you understand it, the more you can anticipate and even prevent some flares before they fully take hold.

Once you start to see those patterns, you can personalize your lifestyle changes to fit your body's specific needs. This doesn't mean overhauling everything overnight — in fact, the most successful changes tend to be small, gradual adjustments that build over time. If you know sun exposure triggers your skin flares, you might make sun protection part of your daily routine, not just something you think about on vacation. If you notice stress makes your fatigue unbearable, you might work meditation, gentle movement, or more scheduled downtime into your week, even before stress piles up. If poor sleep consistently leaves you feeling worse, improving your sleep environment and creating wind-down rituals might become part of your action plan. The key is tailoring these changes to fit your actual life — not someone else's ideal version of self-care. It's not about perfection or following rigid rules, but about working with the body you have, gently adjusting routines and habits to help support your health, rather than fight against it.

Just as important as making changes is setting realistic health goals — goals that fit within the reality of living with a chronic illness. It's easy to set yourself up for frustration if your goals are too ambitious or ignore the unpredictable nature of lupus. A goal like "never have a flare again" might sound good on paper, but it's not realistic — and it sets you up to feel like a failure when the next inevitable flare arrives. Instead, effective health goals focus on things you can control, even in the face of flares. Goals like walking three times a week (as tolerated), staying hydrated, or keeping up with regular follow-ups are both achievable and flexible — they allow for the ups and downs of chronic illness while still giving you a sense of progress and purpose. It's also okay to set goals that have nothing to do with your health — goals for your career, family, hobbies, or travel — because you are not just a lupus patient. Your roadmap should leave space for all parts of you, not just your disease.

Another important piece of your lupus roadmap is learning how to manage life transitions — those moments when your routine, your responsibilities, or your environment changes dramatically. Life doesn't pause for lupus, and big transitions — starting a new job, moving, having a baby, sending your kids off to college — all bring new challenges to how you manage your disease. A personalized action plan doesn't just cover the quiet, stable times — it includes flexibility for the curveballs, whether they come from lupus itself or from life. During transitions, you may need to reassess your medications, add extra self-care practices, or lean more heavily on your support system. Knowing that your plan can adapt with you — that it's not a static list, but a living guide you can update anytime — helps you approach changes with more confidence and less fear.

The beauty of building your own lupus roadmap is that it puts you back in the driver's seat, even in a situation where so much feels out of your control. Your roadmap won't prevent every flare, or erase every bad day, but it gives you structure — a sense of agency — and a framework for making decisions when things feel overwhelming. It's also a reminder that you know your body better than anyone. Doctors bring their expertise, but you bring your lived experience, and when the two come together, the best care happens.

Most of all, your roadmap should be personal and flexible — a reflection of your goals, your limitations, your strengths, and your hopes. It's not a checklist you have to complete perfectly every day, but a guide you can turn to when you need clarity, support, or reassurance that you're still on track, even when lupus throws you off balance. Over time, it becomes not just a plan, but a record of resilience, proof of how you've adapted, grown, and reclaimed control, piece by piece, one flare, one good day, one adjustment at a time. Lupus may be part of your life, but with your own roadmap in hand, it doesn't have to define your path. You are the author of your own story — and this roadmap is how you write the next chapter on your own terms.